EAT LESS SALT

ALSO BY THE AMERICAN HEART ASSOCIATION

American Heart Association Low-Salt Cookbook, 4th Edition
American Heart Association Healthy Slow Cooker Cookbook
American Heart Association Quick & Easy Cookbook, 2nd Edition
American Heart Association No-Fad Diet, 2nd Edition
The New American Heart Association Cookbook, 8th Edition
American Heart Association Quick & Easy Meals
American Heart Association Complete Guide to Women's Heart Health
American Heart Association Healthy Family Meals
American Heart Association Low-Fat, Low-Cholesterol Cookbook, 4th Edition
American Heart Association Low-Calorie Cookbook
American Heart Association One-Dish Meals

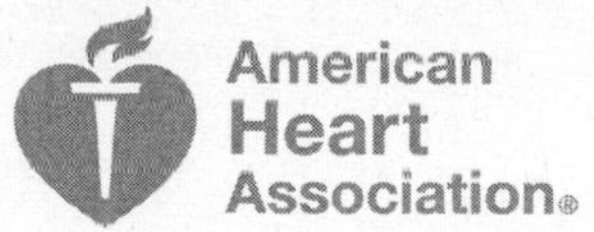

EAT LESS SALT

an easy action plan for finding and reducing the sodium hidden in your diet

with 60 heart-healthy recipes

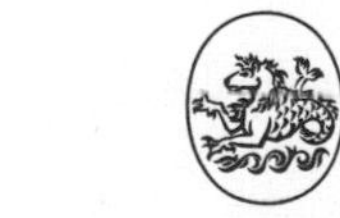

Clarkson Potter/Publishers
New York

No book, including this one, can ever replace the services of a healthcare professional in providing information about your health. You should check with your healthcare professional before using the information in this or any other health-related book. Because numerous variables account for a wide range of values for certain foods, the nutrition analyses for the recipes and the sodium values provided throughout this book should be considered approximate. Different results may be obtained by using different nutrient databases and different brand-name products. The author and the publisher expressly disclaim responsibility for any adverse effects that may result from your use of the information contained in this book.

 Published in the United States by Clarkson Potter/Publishers, an imprint of the Crown Publishing Group, a division of Random House, Inc., New York.
www.crownpublishing.com
www.clarksonpotter.com

Your contributions to the American Heart Association support research that helps make publications like this possible. For more information, call 1-800-AHA-USA1 (1-800-242-8721) or contact us online at www.heart.org.

Library of Congress Cataloging-in-Publication Data
American Heart Association eat less salt.
p. cm.
1. Salt-free diet. I. American Heart Association. II. Title: Eat less salt.
RM237.8.A43 2013
613.2'85223—dc23 2012015399

ISBN 978-0-307-88804-4
eISBN 978-0-307-88805-1

Printed in the United States of America

Book and cover design by Ashley Tucker
Cover photography by Kristin Duvall/Getty Images

10 9 8 7 6 5 4 3 2 1

First Edition

Acknowledgments

AMERICAN HEART ASSOCIATION CONSUMER PUBLICATIONS

DIRECTOR: Linda S. Ball

MANAGING EDITOR: Deborah A. Renza

SENIOR EDITORS: Janice Roth Moss, Robin P. Loveman

SCIENCE EDITOR/WRITER: Jacqueline Fornerod Haigney

ASSISTANT EDITOR: Roberta Westcott Sullivan

RECIPE DEVELOPERS

Ellen Boeke

Nancy S. Hughes

Annie King

Julie Shapero, R.D., L.D.

NUTRITION ANALYST

Tammi Hancock, R.D.

AMERICAN HEART ASSOCIATION SCIENCE AND MEDICINE ADVISOR

Dorothea Vafiadis

Contents

Preface

Most Americans today, including an estimated 97 percent of our children, are eating an unhealthy amount of sodium—and as a result, we have seen the incidence of high blood pressure rise all across the country. In fact, unless this trend changes, nine out of ten Americans may develop high blood pressure at some time in their lives. Scientific evidence shows that eating a high-sodium diet increases the chance that your blood pressure will rise to a dangerous level. To prevent that increase and its potentially deadly effects, we want to do everything possible to help you eat less sodium. We know that our current food supply makes that difficult, but we're here to help!

Because our mission is to reduce the incidence of cardiovascular disease, including stroke, and eliminate its devastating consequences, the American Heart Association is deeply committed to reducing the amount of sodium in the current food supply. We are working with the food industry and government regulatory agencies to join us in this commitment. The American Heart Association has revised its recommendation for daily sodium intake to less than 1,500 milligrams, which is based on scientific research on healthy sodium levels. Sodium is an important part of our diets, but we need only about 500 milligrams per day under normal circumstances. Yet the average American currently consumes about 3,400 milligrams—more than double the amount we recommend for most people. (There are some exceptions to the 1,500-milligram limit, however. For example, people who lose sodium because of environmental conditions, such as working in hot factories or hiking in the desert, and people with medical conditions that cause the body to need more sodium should not restrict their sodium intake to that level.)

We recognize that the task of reducing sodium brings with it many inherent challenges. It isn't easy to change ingrained habits quickly, and the existing food environment presents more highly salted options than it does heart-healthy opportunities. The objective of this book, however, is to help you understand both why it's so important to live a healthy lifestyle *and* how to gradually transition to get to that goal. It's okay to take small steps rather than one big leap—in fact, we recommend it.

Your first step is to acknowledge that doing something to establish a healthier diet is better than doing nothing. Any sodium reduction you make, no matter how small, is a step in the right direction. Once you've made a few meaningful changes in your eating habits, you can choose to move on at your own pace, using the realistic strategies and stair-step approaches this book suggests.

Some of the how-tos you'll find throughout include:

- How to accurately and realistically assess your current sodium intake
- How to reduce the number of high-sodium products in your pantry, refrigerator, and freezer
- How to read food labels
- How to uncover the sodium hidden in foods
- How to keep sodium in line when you eat out
- How to build an overall healthy, lower-sodium diet
- How to create your own personalized healthy menus

We believe that with solid health information, an achievable action plan, and more than 60 heart-healthy versions of popular high-sodium recipes, you can lower your salt intake *and* enjoy the food you eat.

Adopting a lifestyle that supports your lower-sodium goals is necessary for good heart health—and those goals are attainable, one step at a time.

Rose Marie Robertson, M.D.
CHIEF SCIENCE OFFICER
AMERICAN HEART ASSOCIATION/AMERICAN STROKE ASSOCIATION

PART I

Sodium and Your Heart Health

Why has salt, a simple ingredient found on everyone's table, become such a hot topic in the fields of nutrition and health? The explanation is anything *but* simple, yet the facts established after years of research and debate leave little doubt that we are all eating far more sodium in the form of salt than is healthy.

FACT: The more sodium you take in, the higher your blood pressure is likely to be. We know that the connection between sodium and blood pressure is direct and progressive and has no threshold.

FACT: You have a 90 percent chance of developing high blood pressure at some point in your lifetime. More than 75 million people over the age of 20 have high blood pressure today, and that number is growing every day.

FACT: If you have high blood pressure, you are at much higher risk for heart attack, stroke, and other cardiovascular diseases. The effects of high blood pressure can have deadly consequences, especially if left untreated.

FACT: Americans are eating more sodium in the form of processed foods than ever before. Most of us consume almost *seven times* what our bodies need and *more than double* what the American Heart Association recommends for good heart health.

As a nation, this level of excess sodium consumption has put our collective health in jeopardy. Too much sodium means higher blood pressure, which leads to a higher risk of disease and disability. For you as an individual, that connection means that the sooner you reduce the level of sodium in your diet, the better your chances of protecting your heart and preventing heart disease and stroke in your future.

CHAPTER 1

Sodium, Salt, and Our Food Supply

THE BASICS OF SODIUM AND SALT

Many people think of salt and sodium as being the same thing, but they aren't. *Sodium* is a mineral that occurs throughout nature in more than 80 forms. It is the sixth most abundant naturally occurring element on the planet, and it is essential to many of life's functions. In the human body, in particular, sodium is crucial in maintaining the intricate balance of fluids in and around the body's cells, and we can't live without it.

Ninety percent of the sodium we eat comes in the form of salt. *Salt* is a naturally occurring compound that consists of 40 percent sodium and 60 percent chloride. It is found in oceans and salt lakes and in deposits that are the remains of dried-up ancient oceans.

Differences in the techniques used to collect and process salt have created the variety of salts available today. In the grocery store, most of the salts you will find are fine grained, such as regular table salt. (Most table salts are iodized, which means iodine has been added to prevent deficiency in that mineral.) Coarser-grained salts include kosher salt, which is made of large, irregular crystals with a lot of surface area. Sea salt can be either fine or coarse grained, and its flavor and color vary depending on its mineral content.

When it comes to your health, however, the bottom line is that salt is salt. One teaspoon of table salt contains about 2,300 milligrams (mg) of sodium, and all salts contain roughly the same amount regardless of where they come from. It is the quantity of salt you eat that matters—not the kind. No matter how a salt is collected or refined, how it is presented, or how large the crystals, it's still salt, and you must consider the cumulative negative health impact too much of any of these salts can have.

WHERE DOES SALT COME FROM? The oldest and still most common way globally to collect salt is directly from the ocean (sea, or solar, salt). Used for centuries, this technique involves letting salinated water evaporate in large salt pans. In the United States, however, most commercial salt is taken from underground sources, either by injecting water into deposits beneath the surface to create a salty brine that is then processed (evaporated salt), or by using conventional mining to bring the salt to the surface (rock salt). The collected salt is then left unrefined or is ground into fine or coarse grains.

Why We Need Sodium

Our bodies' core systems—circulation, respiration, elimination, and the communication between the brain and the nervous system—depend on a delicate balance between sodium and other chemicals in the body. To maintain the level of sodium in the fluid surrounding the body's cells, the kidneys, endocrine glands, and brain work together continuously to assess and adjust as needed. This balance is so important because any disruption affects the health of every cell, and an estimated 20 to 40 percent of an adult's resting energy is used to maintain it.

Sodium is essential in the intricate processes that generate electrical signals throughout the nervous system, and it regulates how body fluids are distributed and retained—in particular, blood volume and blood pressure. These crucial functions cannot take place without an adequate supply of sodium; however, too much will cause more harm than good.

When So Much Is Too Much

If sodium is so important to our health, how can it become so dangerous? The answer lies in the fact that most of us eat much more sodium than our bodies can handle. Although the exact amount varies for each individual, most people need only about 500 mg of sodium each day to maintain the right balance for their bodies to function properly. *The American Heart Association recommends no more than 1,500 mg of sodium a day, yet the current national average daily intake is about 3,400 mg.*

Over time, the cumulative effects of that much sodium can have devastating health consequences. The human body's mechanisms for conserving the sodium it needs are extremely effective: when sodium is low, the body reacts by conserving water to keep the sodium it has; when sodium levels are too high, the kidneys regulate the level of fluid in the body and flush away the excess sodium in urine. If the kidneys cannot keep pace with the amount of sodium coming in, the body tries to dilute the sodium by retaining water. This leaches water out of the cells into the bloodstream, increasing the volume of fluid in circulation. When blood volume increases, your heart must work harder to pump blood, resulting in higher blood pressure that can stiffen and damage blood vessels and put other body systems under stress.

Unfortunately, these changes usually go undetected until a serious condition, such as high blood pressure, is diagnosed. (The physical effects of sodium excess are covered in more detail in Chapter 2.) There is no doubt, however, that blood pressure rises with higher amounts of dietary sodium and that uncontrolled high blood pressure can cause debilitating cardiovascular problems, including heart disease and stroke. If 90 percent of Americans are likely to develop this potentially deadly condition at some point in their lives, as researchers estimate, it is equally clear that everyone—regardless of age—should take action to reduce the sodium in his or her diet.

SODIUM IN TODAY'S FOOD SUPPLY

Our bodies' biological needs for sodium haven't changed over time, but the ways we eat and how we get our food have changed drastically. Since ancient times, salt has been a valuable resource and has been used for medicinal purposes, as currency, and in food. Salt has always been used both to preserve perishable food and to intensify flavor, which are the same primary reasons salt is used so extensively today. In fact, it is the salt added to foods *before* they reach your table that accounts for the excess of sodium in our food supply.

> **THE IMPORTANCE OF SALT THROUGH HISTORY Salt inhibits the growth of bacteria and fungus, so people found ways to use it to preserve foods that otherwise could not be kept edible for long (e.g., salted fish). Salt was so important in trade and commerce that references to it can be found around the globe, in all languages and from all civilizations. For example, the word *salary* comes from the Latin root *sal*, which means salt. It is said that the Romans valued salt very highly. They originally paid their soldiers with salt rations called "salarium"; when they began to give the soldiers money to buy their own salt, the term stuck.**

Beyond the Saltshaker

Despite the pervasive idea that most of the sodium we consume comes from the saltshaker, very few people add enough table salt to their food to compete with the high levels of sodium found in processed products. According to a study on sodium reduction strategies from the Institute of Medicine, *only 6 percent of the sodium that Americans consume comes from salt added at the table and only 5 percent is added during cooking at home.* Even if you don't sprinkle your food with salt from a shaker at all, you still may be consuming too much sodium. Where, then, is it coming from?

BREAKDOWN OF SODIUM CONSUMPTION

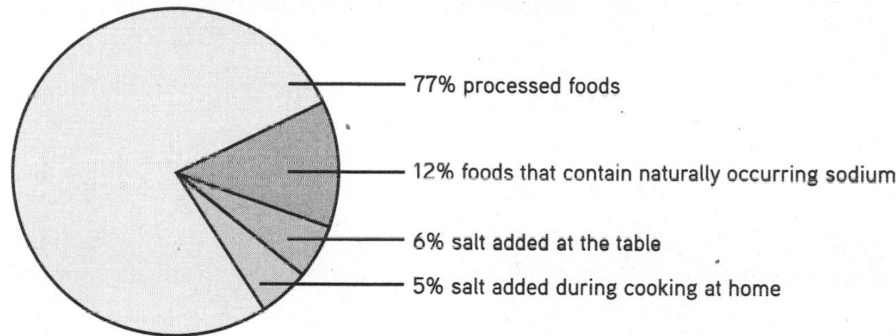

As this chart illustrates, *more than three-quarters of the sodium in our food supply comes from processed foods, including those we eat at restaurants.* Most unprocessed foods contain very little sodium, although there are a few exceptions, such as spinach and celery. In general, however, the nutritional value of these natural foods more than offsets the sodium they contain.

Why then is there so much sodium in processed foods? Manufacturers include salt and sodium additives because they need their products to be attractive and to last without spoiling. The use of salt in various processing techniques helps bind ingredients, improve flavor, and enhance the color of commercial packaged foods. As a result, the amount of added salt in practically every food category has gradually increased in recent years, even in foods that don't taste salty. Restaurants, too, want their dishes to stand out, and a reliable way to pique customers' taste buds and bump up flavor inexpensively is to add more salt.

What does "processed" mean? The term *processed* generally refers to food that isn't eaten directly from the source, such as a plant or an animal. The juice you squeeze directly from an orange, for example, is an unprocessed food. If that juice is commercially prepared and other ingredients are added, such as sugars or preservatives, the resulting orange juice is a processed product. Both the quantity and quality of additives and preservatives, such as salt, can change foods in ways that make them less nutritious. Whether the additives are to heighten flavor, to extend shelf life, or for some other reason, any type of processing will affect the end product.

TOP 10 SOURCES OF SODIUM

1. Breads and rolls
2. Cold cuts and cured meats, such as deli or packaged ham and turkey
3. Pizza
4. Fresh and processed chicken and turkey
5. Soups
6. Sandwiches, including burgers
7. Cheese
8. Pasta dishes with sauce
9. Mixed meat dishes, such as meat loaf with sauce
10. Snacks, such as chips, pretzels, and popcorn

The type of processed food is important, too, because the more often it is part of your diet, the more sodium it contributes. According to data from the Centers for Disease Control and Prevention (CDC), more than 40 percent of the sodium in the average American diet comes from only 10 types of food.

Finding Hidden Sodium

You would expect to find sodium in foods that taste salty, but as the examples in the chart below show, many common foods can be surprisingly high in sodium that is "hidden," or at least not very obvious until you look for it.

FOOD	SODIUM (MG)*	% OF DAILY RECOMMENDATION**
beverages		
energy drink, 8 oz	200	13
tomato juice, 8 oz	655	44
breads		
English muffin, 2 halves	200	13
bagel, 3½ oz, 2 halves	545	36
cereals		
oat rings, 1 cup	160	11
bran flakes, 1½ cups	440	29
condiments		
ketchup, 1 tbsp	170	11
soy sauce, 1 tbsp	1,000	67
dairy products		
low-fat Cheddar cheese, 1 oz	175	12
low-fat cottage cheese, ¾ cup	600	40

*Sodium values have been rounded to the nearest 5 mg.

**American Heart Association Daily Recommendation = 1,500 mg or less.

Be aware that any food that has been processed in some way is likely to contain added sodium. Keep in mind, too, that although a processed food itself may be a seemingly unlikely source of sodium, the amount of sodium in it is not hidden at all. Reading nutrition labels is the best way to find out how much sodium is in the processed foods that you eat.

Many food manufacturers are working to reformulate their products to reduce sodium, but the process is complicated, costly, and time-consuming. Until consumers accept, and adapt to, less salty versions of their favorite foods and demonstrate their preference by asking for and purchasing lower-sodium products at the grocery store, the industry will continue to move carefully.

Why We Like Salty Foods

Some researchers believe that our innate taste for salt dates back to our early survival instincts. They theorize that a sense of taste allowed early humans to decide whether a food was beneficial and safe to eat. For example, sourness or bitterness might have been an indication that a food was spoiled or poisonous, so our ancestors learned to avoid that food. Because humans need to eat adequate amounts of sodium to survive, our ancestors may have learned to identify food that contained sodium by its salty taste. We therefore may be hardwired to detect the taste of salt and find it pleasurable.

On the other hand, many believe that we learn our tolerance for the salty taste from the current level of sodium in our food. When you put food in your mouth, the water in your saliva dissolves chemicals that are detected by the receptor cells located in your taste buds. These receptors send signals to your brain that you are experiencing a "salty" taste. You are born with a low threshold for salt—that is, a threshold at which point overly salted foods begin to taste unpleasant. If you eat a lot of salted food, however, your threshold is raised and you gradually become used to the taste of salt.

The more often you expose your taste receptors to salt, the more they will adjust, or become desensitized, to its flavor. Over time, your taste receptors may need more sodium in food before they register the same level of pleasure in your brain. What you are doing, in essence, is training your taste buds to tolerate more salt than you need.

Scientists are studying how the brain's perception of taste affects eating habits and preferences. One study found that when participants on a lower-sodium diet were allowed to salt the outside of their food, their taste for salt was satisfied even though they were eating less sodium overall than they were used to.

Genetic influences may play a role in why certain people taste sodium more or less intensely than others. Researchers found that some people, called "super-tasters," eat more salty foods than "non-tasters" because super-tasters enjoy the salty taste more and seem to need higher levels of sodium to block out flavors that are unpleasant to them but less obvious to the non-tasters.

Regardless of why we have collectively come to like salty food so much, you can reverse the trend in your own eating habits. By making gradual changes to reduce your intake of sodium, you allow your taste buds to regain their sensitivity. In time—usually between six weeks and six months—you will find that your palate has adjusted and the food you used to enjoy now tastes too salty. In fact, you probably will even notice flavors that have been there all the time but were masked by the salt.

Why We Eat Too Much Salt

In the early 1970s, the average daily sodium intake for American adults was about 2,400 mg. Today's average is about 3,400 mg—1,000 mg more in just one generation. To understand why our intake of sodium has increased so dramatically, we need to look at the changes in both our lifestyle and the modern food supply.

Some of the reasons for this increase lie in the cultural shifts that occurred during those few decades: a faster-paced society with two working parents in many families; more time spent away from home with less time to spend in the kitchen; and a growing desire for fast, convenient foods, including processed foods. As we reallocated how we spent our time, our eating behaviors—how we ate, where we ate, and what we ate—changed, too.

EATING OUT Once saved for a special occasion or treat, eating out has become a favorite American pastime; and when we eat out, the portions likely are large and full of sodium. In fact, it is common for one serving of a typical restaurant entrée to contain twice the amount—or more—of a whole day's worth of sodium, and that's not counting the bread or salad that comes with it. The same can be said of fast-food favorites such as hamburgers, french fries, fried chicken, and pizza—even a "healthy" option such as a salad with dressing. Now that eating out is so prevalent in the U.S. culture, many families eat away from home several times a week—perhaps a time benefit but certainly not a health benefit.

EATING AT HOME Until the last few decades, the typical family ate at home on most nights, with Mom buying and preparing fresh food. Even when convenience products—canned soup, for example—were used, those foods represented a small percentage of what was eaten. Now, however, because of the demands on time and resources, eating at home is not what it once was. Instead of preparing home-cooked meals, many people make food choices based primarily on convenience and cost, and they rely heavily on ready-to-go prepared meals or easy-to-fix packaged foods. When time is short, these shortcuts can be appealing, but the downside is that they can quickly add up to a high-sodium diet. Reading nutrition labels so you know what is in the food you are buying—in particular, sodium, added sugars, and saturated fats—can keep convenience from coming at a cost to your health.

Packaged convenience foods usually contain more sodium—often much more—than their home-cooked counterparts. If you depend on processed foods, those products will be the biggest contributors to your consumption of sodium. If you bought a typical frozen single-serving entrée of turkey breast with gravy, mashed potatoes, and green beans, you could get more than 1,200 mg of sodium. If instead you added some simple gravy to homemade roasted turkey breast, mashed your own potatoes, and steamed some fresh beans, using fresh herbs and salt-free blends as seasonings, you could easily stay below 400 mg. Even if you sprinkled your meal with some salt from your shaker (typically about 1/16 teaspoon), you'd add only 145 mg. That's a savings of about 655 mg for just one meal. You can imagine how quickly your sodium intake can escalate when you eat so much extra sodium at each meal, day after day.

> **ARE SOME SALTS HEALTHIER? Although sea salt and kosher salt are sometimes marketed as more natural and therefore supposedly healthier than regular table salt, all three types contain the same amount of sodium chloride. The differences are that trace amounts of minerals found in sea salt affect taste, and the larger crystals of kosher salt affect texture.**

FOOD MANUFACTURING Economics, too, affects the food choices we make and how manufacturers formulate their products. It is both expensive and difficult, if not impossible, to manufacture certain foods, such as cheese, without using salt. When foods that are now processed foods, such as our cheese example, were made by hand, they were relatively expensive, so few people could afford to eat much of them. As production became more efficient, faster, and more cost-effective, the cheese became more affordable and more widely available. As a result, people are eating more high-sodium cheese than ever before, and few inexpensive low-sodium options are available.

Additionally, when manufacturers reformulate their foods to address a health concern—for instance, reducing the fat in cheese—they need to compensate by adding something to pump up the flavor. Salt, fats, and sugars are inexpensive, enhance flavor, and provide desired tastes, so they become the typical replacements that food companies rely on to make their products more appealing. In the cheese example on page 19, when the fat is reduced, salt or sugars are likely to be increased. The catch-22 result can be a lower-fat but higher-sodium cheese.

Finally, the shelf life of processed foods is much longer than that of most unprocessed foods, resulting in less spoilage and waste in transit for the manufacturer, on store shelves, and in your kitchen. All these changes in the food industry combined with the shifts in the economy and our behaviors have shaped trends that have led to higher amounts of sodium in the American diet, resulting in unintended yet harmful consequences to our health.

The adverse effects of too much sodium, including high blood pressure and heart disease, are too significant to ignore. To protect yourself and your family, you can control the sodium you consume by carefully choosing the foods you eat. You can also make your voice heard by asking for lower-sodium options at the store and in restaurants and by advocating for stricter sodium guidelines for our food supply. Every step you take, big or small, ultimately can have a huge positive impact on your heart health.

CHAPTER 2

Sodium, High Blood Pressure, and Heart Disease

The progression from a high-sodium diet to high blood pressure to increased risk for heart disease and stroke is reflected in the public health statistics. Numbers can be dry reading, but when they are as important as the ones here, they bear both reading and heeding: *one in three U.S. adults currently suffers from high blood pressure,* and predictions estimate that that number will continue to increase. Currently, nearly 350,000 deaths each year are attributed to high blood pressure, yet of all the people with this condition, more than 20 percent are unaware of it. Even among people who do know, 30 percent don't keep their high blood pressure under control.

Contrary to popular belief, high blood pressure does not occur only in people who are middle-aged and older; in fact, no one is immune to it. Although blood pressure usually increases as we age, youth is not a guaranteed antidote—even babies can have high blood pressure. The incidence of this disease in children and young people is increasing, with serious health consequences. Teenagers who have high blood pressure and are obese may develop thickened artery walls by age 30, as well as the arterial fatty buildup that can lead to heart disease and stroke. Sadly, most incidences of high blood pressure in teens and young adults are preventable, because they usually result from an unhealthy lifestyle, including a diet that is too high in sodium.

Even if you don't have high blood pressure now, chances are that you will develop the condition at some point. You can lower your risk, however, by cutting back on the sodium in your diet. Blood pressure begins to decrease for most people within a few weeks of lowering sodium intake, and in most cases, lower blood pressure means reduced risk for cardiovascular disease.

Scientific evidence indicates that for many people, a high-sodium diet increases blood pressure. We also know that untreated high blood pressure is a leading contributor to heart disease and stroke, which together kill one of every three adults in the United States. These grim statistics illustrate just how important it is to understand what blood pressure is and how much it affects your health.

THE BASICS OF BLOOD PRESSURE

To deliver oxygen and nutrients to the body's cells, the heart pumps blood through the circulatory system, a complex network of arteries, capillaries, and veins. Blood pressure is the force of blood as it moves through this system. It is measured as both the pressure exerted against an artery wall when the heart contracts, called systolic pressure, and the pressure in the artery when the heart is at rest between beats, called diastolic pressure. Reported in millimeters of mercury (mmHg), these values are shown as systolic over diastolic pressure, so the readings are given as a fraction—for example, 120/80 mmHg, often referred to simply as 120 over 80.

What Is High Blood Pressure?

When blood pressure is high, more pressure than usual is exerted on the artery walls. This extra pressure damages the smooth lining of the arteries and makes it easier for cholesterol and fat to build up along the artery walls. As the arteries become clogged with fatty layers, less blood gets through and the heart must beat harder as it tries to pump blood through narrowed arteries.

A common misconception is that when your blood pressure is high, you always feel tense, nervous, or hyperactive. Actually, blood pressure has nothing to do with these reactions. In fact, you can feel fine and be relaxed, yet still have high blood pressure. Because high blood pressure usually has no symptoms, and therefore its harmful effects can go unnoticed for years, it is referred to as the "silent killer."

KNOW YOUR BLOOD PRESSURE LEVEL The only way to know your blood pressure level is to have it checked with a blood pressure monitor. All adults—even those with no previous problems—should have their blood pressure checked at least once every two years. People at risk, such as those with a family history of high blood pressure, stroke, or heart attack, need to have it checked more frequently. Children should have their blood pressure checked annually.

Blood pressure falls into three categories: normal, prehypertension, and hypertension. Blood pressure with a systolic pressure less than 120 mmHg *and* diastolic less than 80 mmHg is defined as normal. Slightly elevated blood pressure approaching unhealthful limits is referred to as prehypertension. Blood pressure that measures over 140/90 mmHg on two separate occasions is classified as high, or hypertension.

BLOOD PRESSURE LEVEL*	SYSTOLIC (MMHG)		DIASTOLIC (MMHG)
normal	less than 120	*and*	less than 80
prehypertension	120 to 139	*or*	80 to 89
hypertension	140 or greater	*or*	90 or greater

***For adults 18 years or older. These levels apply only to people who are not taking medication for high blood pressure and who do not have a short-term serious illness.**

In children, a normal reading for blood pressure depends on gender, age, and height. Check with your healthcare professional to learn what is considered healthy for your child.

What Causes High Blood Pressure?

The direct cause of high blood pressure is not known. For many people, however, the risk is increased because of unhealthy habits, including:

- Eating a lot of high-sodium foods
- Consuming too many calories, leading to being overweight or obese
- Not getting enough exercise
- Smoking tobacco or being exposed to secondhand smoke
- Drinking excessive amounts of alcohol

All these lifestyle choices are within your control. In Part II, "Strategies for a Lower-Sodium Lifestyle," you'll learn more about how to target the high-sodium foods in your current diet and live healthier.

Who Is at Risk for High Blood Pressure?

Everyone is at risk for developing high blood pressure at some point. Because of factors that are beyond their control, including race, age, and family history, some people are more at risk than others. For example, more than 40 percent of African American adults have high blood pressure, which may be linked to genetic factors. In particular, blacks, middle-aged and older adults, and people with blood relatives who have or had high blood pressure, as well as people who already have high blood pressure, will benefit from reducing their sodium intake. Unfortunately, there is no test to determine who is more prone to risk of high blood pressure or who will respond to a greater or lesser extent to reducing dietary sodium. The best way for you to stay aware of your risk, then, is to know your blood pressure level and monitor it regularly.

HOW BLOOD PRESSURE AFFECTS HEALTH

To illustrate how increased blood pressure can affect your circulatory system, imagine your blood flowing like a river, traveling through blood vessels from your heart to the rest of your body and back again. When stormy weather turns the usually calm flow of a river into a flood, the rushing water becomes destructive, ruining levees and damaging the riverbanks on either side. When blood pressure is higher than normal, the resulting force of blood crashing against artery walls is like the excessive force of floodwater. In both cases, when such volatile forces continue over time, the consistent pounding can cause permanent damage. The risk factors, or "storms," that can bring on a lasting rise in blood pressure include increasing age, smoking, lack of exercise, excessive use of alcohol, and unhealthy eating habits, especially eating a high-sodium diet. In turn, high blood pressure then greatly increases the risk of heart disease and stroke.

Healthy arteries are made of muscle and elastic tissue that stretch when the heart pumps blood through them. The more forcefully the blood pumps, the more the arteries must stretch to allow it to flow. Over time, if artery walls continually get stretched beyond a healthy limit, the tissue will thicken, lose elasticity, and become damaged.

These changes cause serious problems throughout the circulatory system that compromise heart health and lead to disease. For example:

- Overstretching creates *weaknesses in the smooth linings of blood vessel walls.* These weakened spots are then more prone to rupture, which causes strokes and aneurysms.

- Overstretching also causes tiny tears in the smooth linings, leaving *scar tissue on the walls of arteries and veins.* These tears and scar tissue act like nets, catching blood cells and cholesterol traveling in the bloodstream. Gradually this buildup forms into hard, waxy plaque on vessel walls (atherosclerosis).
- As plaque builds up and narrows the blood vessels, *blood flow is restricted, creating increased pressure* throughout the rest of the circulatory system. As the flow becomes more restricted, the heart must work harder to deliver oxygenated blood throughout the body.
- The increased workload caused by such narrowing and the loss of elasticity can result in *damage to the heart muscles and valves.* As the heart works harder, it also grows larger, and the heavy workload eventually takes its toll by weakening the heart so it cannot pump effectively; that, in turn, leads to heart failure.
- Higher blood pressure increases the risk of *blood clots that break loose and block blood vessels.* Especially when vessels are already narrowed by the buildup of plaque, these clots can block the supply of oxygenated blood to different parts of the body. If the blockage stops blood flowing to the heart, it causes a heart attack. If the blood stops flowing to the brain, it causes a stroke.
- When blood flow is reduced because arteries and veins are narrowed, the circulatory system cannot provide an adequate supply of oxygenated blood, resulting in *damage to tissues and organs.*

What Happens When High Blood Pressure Is Left Untreated

There is no acceptable level of high blood pressure. The consequences of uncontrolled high blood pressure are life-threatening. When this disease goes untreated, it can permanently damage your heart, brain, eyes, and kidneys. It can also lead to heart attack, heart failure, stroke, kidney failure, and other serious events. Evidence also has shown that adults with high blood pressure who smoke, have high blood cholesterol levels, or have diabetes are at even higher risk of heart disease and stroke. Some of the major cardiovascular problems caused by high blood pressure are:

- **CORONARY ARTERY DISEASE.** The coronary arteries supply the heart muscle with oxygen and nutrients. When this blood supply is reduced because of narrowed arteries, so is the supply of oxygen to the heart.

This lack of oxygen causes chest pain, or angina, and increases the risk for heart attack.

- **HEART FAILURE.** When the heart is too weak to pump blood effectively, it must pump more often. At the same time, the kidneys act to increase blood volume by retaining sodium, thus causing even more work for the weak heart. As blood flow out of the heart is reduced, blood returning to the heart through the veins backs up. This causes congestion in body tissues and sometimes accumulation of fluid, particularly in the lungs and legs (termed "congestive heart failure").
- **CARDIOMYOPATHY.** This serious condition affects the heart muscle itself, weakening it so it cannot pump effectively.
- **PERIPHERAL ARTERY DISEASE.** When blood flow to the kidneys, stomach, arms, legs, and feet is restricted, tissues are deprived of oxygen. This results in painful cramping or fatigue in the hips, thighs, and calves during exercise.
- **STROKE.** High blood pressure can damage arteries throughout the body, including the brain. Ischemic strokes occur when arteries in the brain become narrowed or clogged and cut off blood flow to brain cells. High blood pressure can also weaken arterial walls in the brain that may rupture in or near the brain, causing a hemorrhagic stroke.
- **KIDNEY DISEASE.** High blood pressure can cause the arteries around the kidneys to narrow, weaken, or harden over time, depriving the kidney tissue of oxygen and nutrients. The kidneys lose their ability to filter blood and regulate fluids in the body. As more arteries become blocked and stop functioning, the kidneys eventually fail.

HEALTHY EATING IMPROVES BLOOD PRESSURE

The facts are clear: Americans are eating too much sodium, and sodium has a direct impact on blood pressure. The populations of many non-Western countries around the world consume diets low in salt and do not in their later years experience the increase in blood pressure that is seen in most Western countries. If you start to focus on eating a nutritious, lower-sodium diet now, however, you may be able to protect and even improve your heart health as you age by controlling your blood pressure.

The American Heart Association recommends a balanced, varied diet that is rich in minerals and fiber and low in sodium, saturated fat, trans fat, cholesterol, and added sugars. Studies have shown that people, especially African Americans, who adopt a sensible eating pattern and effectively balance the calories they eat with the calories they burn can decrease their blood pressure levels; if they also reduce their sodium intake, their blood pressure drops even more. One DASH (Dietary Approaches to Stop Hypertension) study showed that the less sodium people consumed, the lower their blood pressure, and that backing off salt reduced blood pressure even in those who had normal pressure. Another study found that people who were prehypertensive and cut back on sodium intake reduced their chances of developing cardiovascular disease by 25 percent and their risk of dying from it by 20 percent.

So, how does a healthy diet have such a powerful effect on blood pressure? The keystones in keeping blood pressure in check are:

- Reducing the amount of sodium in your overall diet
- Eating the recommended amounts and combinations of nutrient-rich foods that are right for you, based on your age, height, and activity level

Other important factors may be due to the ways the essential nutrients and minerals in whole foods work together in the body. With its emphasis on a variety of nutrient-rich foods, a heart-healthy diet provides the right combination of enough key elements—especially potassium, calcium, magnesium, and fiber—to consistently lower blood pressure. Conversely, there is good evidence that *not* eating enough of these nutrients may lead to increased blood pressure. Chapter 7, "Stay Focused on Eating Well," details how you can establish a healthy diet that both lowers sodium and provides the rich nutritional value you get from a broad spectrum of food groups.

Whether you are young or old, whether you inherited genes from a father who died of a heart attack at 50 or who lived to be 100, you are at risk of having high blood pressure, especially if you don't control and manage harmful lifestyle habits, such as eating a diet with too much sodium. Each action you take to reduce the sodium in your diet is an important step toward better health. By keeping your sodium intake low and your blood pressure under control, you can significantly minimize your risk of heart disease and maximize your chances of living a longer, healthier life.

PART II

Strategies for a Lower-Sodium Lifestyle

Despite the recent attention given to the high level of sodium in our food supply, a lot of people still don't believe the problem relates to them. When they read reports on the rising incidence of high blood pressure and other heart-related issues, they think, "That's about old people, not about me. I don't have high blood pressure." The truth, however, is that too much sodium poses a health threat for *everyone,* including you, no matter your age, ethnicity, or health.

The first thing to learn about sodium is that *you* can control *it* instead of letting it control your health. After all, you are the one who decides what you will eat, and that puts you in charge of deciding how much of your diet will be high in sodium. Let your individual preferences and health goals drive your choices.

You don't have to kick the high-sodium habit all at once. In fact, given the current food supply and social environment, it's best to take a stepwise approach. The following proven strategies will help you make a realistic transition to a lower-sodium diet.

- **EDUCATE YOURSELF.** (Chapter 3) Learn how to find the amount of sodium in all the foods you eat and assess how sodium adds up in your own diet.
- **START WITH SMALL CHANGES.** (Chapter 4) Identify the patterns and pitfalls in your eating habits, then find ways to review, rethink, and reduce your sodium intake.
- **TARGET HIGH-SODIUM FOODS AT HOME.** (Chapter 5) Find the high-sodium foods you buy regularly and replace them with lower-sodium alternatives.
- **IDENTIFY HIGH-SODIUM FOODS WHEN EATING OUT.** (Chapter 6) Know the sodium levels in your favorite restaurant meals, compare options, and make better choices.
- **STAY FOCUSED ON EATING WELL.** (Chapter 7) Make eating a balanced, heart-smart diet part of your lifestyle.
- **PLAN AHEAD WITH LOWER-SODIUM MENUS.** (Chapter 8) Create delicious and nutritious meals every day—and keep your sodium intake in check.

CHAPTER 3

Educate Yourself

Eating less sodium means having better health, but making that happen isn't as simple as saying that you'll never use a saltshaker again. Because most of the sodium in your diet comes from the salt in prepared and packaged foods, your first step is educating yourself about some important sodium basics: which common foods are typically high in sodium, which specific high-sodium foods you eat often, and how much sodium you consume on average. Once you know those things, you will be prepared to adopt a lower-sodium lifestyle, one step at a time.

SODIUM SHAKEDOWN STRATEGIES

✓ Learn how to read food labels and nutrition facts panels.

✓ Research restaurant menus to find out how much sodium is in your favorite dishes.

✓ Track your *actual* sodium intake by recording the value of everything you consume for one week, and compare your daily average intake to the American Heart Association recommended goal of 1,500 mg or less a day.

✓ Get your blood pressure checked at least once every two years (more often if you are at risk) and keep a record of the results.

TEST YOUR SODIUM SMARTS

With so many foods available and new products appearing every day, it's not easy to know exactly what you are eating at all times. It's natural to assume that a "healthy" food such as salad or cereal should be good for you, but if you want to lower your sodium, you need to be sure your assumptions are correct. Studies show that most people significantly *under*estimate the amount of sodium in both individual foods and their own diets. To find out how well you estimate the sodium, take this quick quiz.

Of these three sample diets for a typical day, which would you guess has the highest sodium content? In each case, you can assume that the amounts consumed are no more than an average serving.

1. *Christy, a 36-year-old stay-at-home mom:* Married with two young children, volunteers at school, pays a lot of attention to what her kids eat, cooks at home as often as possible, and occasionally has a drink with the neighbors.

   Breakfast: Whole-grain cereal with fat-free milk and banana slices
   Lunch: Sandwich of rye bread, deli honey-baked ham, lettuce, tomato, and mustard
   Snack: Organic whole-wheat crackers and Cheddar cheese
   Dinner: Homemade meat loaf, organic brown rice pilaf from a mix, organic canned green beans, salad with homemade vinaigrette (with a pinch of salt), instant sugar-free chocolate pudding
   Beverages: 3 bottled green teas and a frozen margarita with salted rim

2. *Owen, a 54-year-old salesman:* Married with three teenagers, spends most of his time on the road for business, and often eats in restaurants.

   Breakfast: Fried-egg special including hash brown potatoes, buttered toast, and bacon at a hotel restaurant
   Lunch: Cobb salad with grilled chicken and Caesar dressing at a quick-casual restaurant
   Snack: Protein bar
   Dinner: Grilled salmon entrée with steamed broccoli, French bread, and cheesecake while entertaining a client at a high-end restaurant
   Beverages: Orange juice, black coffee, iced tea, a martini, and 2 glasses of white wine

3. *Dan, a 27-year-old construction supervisor:* Unmarried with no children, works outside, plays sports, and eats on the run or has dinner out with friends.

   Breakfast: Egg-and-sausage biscuit sandwich from a convenience store
   Lunch: Fast-food fried fish sandwich with tartar sauce and french fries
   Dinner: Chips and salsa, 3 beef enchiladas, refried beans, and rice at a local Mexican restaurant
   Beverages: Black coffee, 2 colas, an energy drink, water, and 3 beers

4. *Dorothy, a 63-year-old retired teacher:* Divorced with one grown child, lives alone, and is worried about her weight.

   Breakfast: English muffin with light tub margarine, cantaloupe wedge
   Lunch: Consommé, low-fat cottage cheese with salsa, melba toast
   Snack: Celery ribs with peanut butter
   Dinner: Frozen low-calorie Swedish meatballs, frozen seasoned veggie mix, diet-brand fat-free ice cream sandwich
   Snack: Light microwave popcorn
   Beverages: Hot tea with fat-free milk, 2 mixed-vegetable juices

Now look at the actual sodium count for each of these people to see if your assumptions match reality.

1. CHRISTY, THE STAY-AT-HOME MOM

FOODS AND BEVERAGES	SERVING SIZE	SODIUM (MG)*
breakfast		
whole-grain cereal with	1 cup	290
milk, fat-free	4 oz	50
banana slices	½ medium	0
	subtotal	**340**
lunch		
sandwich of		
rye bread	2 slices	400
ham, deli honey-baked, 97% fat-free	2 oz	690
lettuce	3 leaves	0
tomato	2 slices	0
mustard, yellow	2 tsp	115
	subtotal	**1,205**
snack		
organic whole-wheat crackers	6	225
Vermont Cheddar cheese	2 oz	350
	subtotal	**575**
dinner		
homemade meat loaf	4 oz	540
organic brown rice pilaf from a mix	½ cup	530
organic green beans, canned	½ cup	380
salad with	2 cups	40
homemade vinaigrette (with a pinch of salt)	¼ cup	260
instant sugar-free pudding, chocolate	½ cup	420
	subtotal	**2,170**
beverages		
green tea with ginseng, bottled	3 x 8 oz	60
frozen margarita rimmed with salt	6 oz	960
	subtotal	**1,020**
	total	**5,310**

***Sodium values have been rounded to the nearest 5 mg.**

2. OWEN, THE SALESMAN

FOODS AND BEVERAGES	SERVING SIZE	SODIUM (MG)*
breakfast		
fried egg plate with hash brown potatoes and buttered toast	restaurant portion	1,380
bacon	2 strips	300
	subtotal	**1,680**
lunch		
Cobb salad with grilled chicken and Caesar dressing	restaurant portion	**1,130**
snack		
protein bar, peanut butter	1 bar	**200**
dinner		
grilled salmon with steamed broccoli	restaurant portion	1,240
French bread	1 slice	160
lemon cheesecake	1 large slice	420
	subtotal	**1,820**
beverages		
orange juice, fresh	8 oz	0
coffee, black	8 oz	0
iced tea, unsweetened	12 oz	0
martini with 2 green olives	6 oz	370
white wine	2 x 4 oz	10
	subtotal	**380**
	total	5,210

*Sodium values have been rounded to the nearest 5 mg.

3. DAN, THE CONSTRUCTION SUPERVISOR

FOODS AND BEVERAGES	SERVING SIZE	SODIUM (MG)*
breakfast		
egg-and-sausage biscuit sandwich from convenience store	fast-food portion	**1,210**
lunch		
fried fish sandwich with tartar sauce	restaurant portion	1,050
french fries	3 oz	350
	subtotal	**1,400**
dinner		
chips with	2 oz	240
salsa	2 tbsp	220
beef enchiladas	3	730
refried beans	½ cup	560
Mexican rice	½ cup	530
	subtotal	**2,280**
beverages		
coffee, black	8 oz	0
cola	2 x 12 oz	100
energy drink	8 oz	200
beer	3 x 12 oz	30
	subtotal	**330**
	total	5,220

***Sodium values have been rounded to the nearest 5 mg.**

4. DOROTHY, THE RETIRED TEACHER

FOODS AND BEVERAGES	SERVING SIZE	SODIUM (MG)*
breakfast		
English muffin with	1 muffin	200
light tub margarine	1 tbsp	105
cantaloupe	1 small wedge	10
	subtotal	**315**
lunch		
consommé, canned	½ cup	810
cottage cheese, low-fat, with	¾ cup	600
salsa	¼ cup	460
melba toast	4 pieces	120
	subtotal	**1,990**
snack		
celery ribs with	4 medium	200
peanut butter	¼ cup	300
	subtotal	**500**
dinner		
frozen Swedish meatballs, low-calorie entrée	10 oz	710
frozen seasoned vegetable mix	¾ cup	260
ice cream sandwich, fat-free	1 sandwich	150
	subtotal	**1,120**
snack		
microwave popcorn, light	6 cups popped	**220**
beverages		
hot tea with	6 oz	0
milk, fat-free	1 oz	15
mixed-vegetable juice	2 x 8 oz	720
	subtotal	**735**
	total	4,880

*Sodium values have been rounded to the nearest 5 mg.

Now, take a few minutes to think about the following:

- Are you surprised at how much sodium each person is eating or by who is eating the most?
- Did you expect one of the lifestyles to lead to a sodium level that was lower or higher than the others?
- Most important, do you recognize yourself in any of these scenarios?

The truth is that almost everyone's diet is too high in sodium. That's why it is so important to make the effort to learn about what you eat and drink.

Sodium has a way of sneaking up on you. It's pretty obvious that salty-tasting foods, such as pretzels and french fries, contain sodium, but it's not so easy to detect the salt in many other popular foods. To test your sodium savvy for individual foods, choose the higher-sodium food from each pair below. (Both options are of similar weight.) The answers follow on pages 37–38.

1. **a.** 1 large slice of raisin bread
b. 1 small slice of French bread

2. **a.** 1 ounce processed low-fat American cheese
b. 1 ounce processed low-fat Swiss cheese

3. **a.** ¼ cup pancake syrup
b. ¼ cup pure maple syrup

4. **a.** 1 cup raisin bran
b. 1 cinnamon-raisin English muffin

5. **a.** 1 ounce plain salted potato chips
b. 1 ounce plain salted pretzels

6. **a.** 2 tablespoons low-fat Italian dressing
b. 2 tablespoons low-fat ranch dressing

7. **a.** 2 (1-ounce) slices regular deli honey-baked ham
b. 2 (1-ounce) slices oven-roasted deli turkey breast

8. **a.** ½ cup marinara sauce
b. ½ cup Alfredo sauce

9. **a.** 1 cup prepared condensed tomato soup
b. 1 cup prepared condensed chicken noodle soup

10. **a.** 1 tablespoon soy sauce
b. 1 tablespoon teriyaki sauce

ANSWERS

1. A 2-inch slice of French bread **(b)** contains about 160 mg of sodium, compared with 125 in one slice of raisin bread. Salt is added to most breads to control the rising action of the dough and to improve texture, but the amount can vary widely among brands. Always check the nutrition facts panels when buying breads and muffins, and choose the lower-sodium options.

2. The low-fat American cheese **(a)** is much higher, containing an average of 430 mg of sodium, than the Swiss cheese at only 75 mg. Making cheese requires some salt, but there is a lot of variation in processing methods. In general, the more highly processed the cheese, the higher the sodium.

3. The processed pancake syrup **(a)** has about 55 mg of sodium, compared with only 10 mg in the pure maple syrup.

4. Sweet raisin bran **(a)** can contain 250 to 340 mg of sodium per cup, making the English muffin the lower-sodium choice at 200 mg. Salt is added to enhance flavors, so even though a cereal tastes sugary sweet, it often contains a great deal of sodium as well.

5. The pretzels **(b)** have more sodium, about 500 mg, than the potato chips at an average of 170 mg. Why? Like breads, pretzel dough contains salt, and more salt is added after baking. Even unsalted pretzels typically contain 80 to 100 mg—more sodium than you might expect. For a lower-sodium pretzel, try the recipe on page 196.

6. Italian dressing **(a)** can add between 300 and 510 mg of sodium to salad greens. Ranch dressing contains less, averaging between 150 and 370 mg, but that is still considered high for a 2-tablespoon portion. The typical commercial salad dressing is high in sodium, so it pays to compare labels when shopping. If you make your dressings, it is easy to control the sodium level. For suggestions, see the recipes on pages 224–226.

7. The ham **(a)** is higher at 690 mg for only two slices, or about 2 ounces. The same amount of turkey is a lower-sodium choice at about 500 mg. However, all processed meats are high in sodium because salt is used in the curing or is added as a preservative. To support your cardiovascular health, the American Heart Association recommends that you eat no more than two servings a week of processed meats. Instead of store-bought deli meats, try one of the recipes for roast beef and roasted poultry on pages 150 and 160.

8. A half cup of Alfredo sauce **(b)** will add 640 to 980 mg of sodium to pasta; an equal amount of marinara ranges from 220 to 780 mg. Commercial pasta sauce is another product that varies widely in sodium content, so always read the nutrition facts panels and choose the lowest-sodium sauces you can find. However, making your own sauces, such as the ones on pages 213 and 215, is the best way to control the sodium.

9. One cup of prepared condensed chicken noodle soup **(b)** has more sodium at 890 mg—more than half a day's worth. Tomato soup can vary from 480 to 890 or more mg, depending on the brand. Canned and packaged soups have been notoriously high in sodium, but food manufacturers are now making many lower-sodium options. Be sure to keep checking labels and looking for new products, and heed the serving sizes listed. Better yet, it's easy to make your own lower-sodium soups. You also might want to prepare large batches of different broths to keep in the freezer so you will have a ready supply to use as the base of many soups and as flavoring for a wide variety of other dishes (see recipes on pages 174–184).

10. Salty-tasting soy sauce **(a)** wins the highest-sodium award of all the foods mentioned in this quiz, on average coming in at a whopping 1,000 mg *in each tablespoon*. Teriyaki contains between 390 and 690 mg, but that certainly doesn't qualify it as a low-sodium choice! The sodium in condiments can really add up, so it's important to choose the brands that are lowest and then to watch how much you use.

NOTE: The values used here represent averages of "regular" or "traditional" versions of widely available packaged foods. The data come from the U.S. Department of Agriculture (USDA) National Nutrient Database for Standard Reference, which averages the nutrient values of multiple commercially prepared food products of the same type.

How did you do? What surprised you? To get the lowdown on sodium and raise your score, keep reading. The more you know about nutrition facts and sodium, the better equipped you will be to make smarter decisions.

LEARN THE FACTS

Because so much of the food we eat these days is processed and commercially distributed, your primary go-to resource to find sodium information is the nutrition labeling on food packaging. You may already be used to checking nutrition labeling for calories when you shop. If so, retrain your brain and make the sodium value a priority, too.

Compare Labels on Packaged Foods

For almost all manufactured food, the nutrition facts panel on the package will tell you the amount of nutrients, including sodium, in one serving of that food. The U.S. Food and Drug Administration (FDA) and the USDA regulate the information that's listed on the panel, so you can compare products and understand what you are buying.

Depending on the manufacturer's brand and the preparation, the sodium content in similar processed foods can vary a lot. In the following example, when you compare the labels of frozen green peas and canned peas side by side, it's easy to see that the canned peas contain three times as much sodium.

Frozen Peas

Nutrition Facts	
Serving Size 1 cup	
Servings Per Container About 3	
Amount Per Serving	
Calories 60	Calories from Fat 0
	% Daily Value*
Total Fat 0g	0%
Saturated Fat 0g	0%
Trans Fat 0g	
Cholesterol 0mg	0%
Sodium 125mg	5%
Total Carbohydrate 11g	4%
Dietary Fiber 6g	22%
Sugars 5g	
Protein 5g	
Vitamin A 15%	Vitamin C 30%
Calcium 0%	Iron 6%

*Percent Daily Values are based on a 2,000-calorie diet. Your daily values may be higher or lower depending on your calorie needs.

Canned Peas

Nutrition Facts	
Serving Size 1 cup	
Servings Per Container About 3	
Amount Per Serving	
Calories 60	Calories from Fat 0
	% Daily Value*
Total Fat 0g	0%
Saturated Fat 0g	0%
Trans Fat 0g	
Cholesterol 0mg	0%
Sodium 380mg	16%
Total Carbohydrate 12g	4%
Dietary Fiber 3g	14%
Sugars 4g	
Protein 4g	
Vitamin A 6%	Vitamin C 10%
Calcium 2%	Iron 8%

*Percent Daily Values are based on a 2,000-calorie diet. Your daily values may be higher or lower depending on your calorie needs.

WATCH OUT FOR PORTION DISTORTION When you're shopping for food, size matters. As you check the nutrition facts panel for the sodium value, be sure to also take note of the serving size, which can be a real blind spot. Unless you're comparing equivalent amounts of a product, the choice you make can be way off. Pasta sauce is a great example of how much variance you'll find among brands and types. Not only do ingredients and flavors differ, but many times so does the serving size. When you find yourself comparing sodium levels for products that don't use similar serving sizes, you will need to do some simple math to calculate equivalent amounts of the product to be sure you are getting an accurate idea of which is the better option. For example, if you glance quickly at the nutrition label on a typical jar of marinara sauce, you'll see that the sodium reads 510 mg. Check the label on a jar of Alfredo sauce and it will read about 410 mg. Yet if you read the labels carefully, you'll see that the serving size of Alfredo sauce is ¼ cup, or *half* that of the marinara, so its comparable sodium content in ½ cup is actually 820 mg. When you do the math, it's easy to see that the Alfredo is the much higher-sodium choice.

Alfredo Sauce

Nutrition Facts	
Serving Size ¼ cup	
Servings Per Container About 7	
Amount Per Serving	
Calories 100	Calories from Fat 80
	% Daily Value*
Total Fat 9g	14%
Saturated Fat 5g	25%
Trans Fat 0g	0%
Cholesterol 50mg	17%
Sodium 410mg	17%

Marinara Sauce

Nutrition Facts	
Serving Size ½ cup	
Servings Per Container About 5	
Amount Per Serving	
Calories 70	Calories from Fat 20
	% Daily Value*
Total Fat 2g	3%
Saturated Fat 0g	0%
Trans Fat 0g	0%
Cholesterol 0mg	0%
Sodium 510mg	21%

KNOW THE SODIUM SPECIFICS Manufacturers are required to use specific phrases if they want to describe the sodium content of their foods. Each has a meaning defined by the FDA and the USDA.

- "Sodium free" means 5 mg of sodium or less per serving.
- "Very low sodium" means 35 mg of sodium or less per serving.
- "Low sodium" means 140 mg of sodium or less per serving.
- "Reduced sodium" means at least 25 percent less sodium than in the original version. (Be aware, however, that many reduced-sodium foods, such as chicken broth, soups, and soy sauce, still contain significant amounts of sodium.)
- "Unsalted" or "no salt added" means no salt was added during processing. (This does not necessarily mean, however, that the product is sodium free.)

These terms refer only to sodium content. Remember that although foods may have little if any sodium, they may be high in calories, saturated fat, trans fat, and/or cholesterol.

CHECK OUT HEALTH CLAIMS Watch out for packaging that is designed to present a "healthy" image. Claim-based icons and terms such as "heart-smart" or "healthy" may make a product seem like a better bet, but you can't assume that these claims mean low sodium. The FDA allows manufacturers to advertise claims based on specific rules for the particular nutritional element. For example, a label on a packaged food may accurately claim that the food is low in saturated fat or cholesterol, but you won't know whether it is also low in sodium unless you read the label. Although foods labeled "all natural," "organic," "gluten free," or "low fat" may provide some benefit that appeals to you, remember that these products can also be high in sodium. Your best bet is to question the front-of-package *marketing* messages and rely on the *nutrition facts* label for information.

AIM FOR ACCEPTABLE AMOUNTS When shopping to keep your sodium low, look for foods that fall within an established "acceptable range" for that category. Decide in advance what your personal limits are for different types of foods and beverages, then look at the numbers in the left column on the nutrition facts panel to see exactly how many milligrams of sodium that food contains. For example, you could decide to choose entrées that contain less than 400 mg per serving, and for most other categories, you could look for items that have less than 140 mg per serving. The numbers in the right column—the % Daily Value (DV)—represent the percentage of each nutrient in a single serving, in terms of the daily recommended amount. If you want to consume less sodium, choose foods with a lower % Daily Value; 5% or less is considered low. (If you want to consume more of a beneficial nutrient, such as fiber, look for foods with a higher % Daily Value; 20% or more is considered high.)

UNDERSTAND ADDITIVES Sodium in processed foods doesn't always come in the form of salt. Sodium is often added to foods and medicines in forms that are not easily recognized. When reading ingredient lists, you may come across the names of the common sodium-adding ingredients listed on the next page (we also included their commercial uses).

SODIUM ADDITIVE	USE
Baking soda; baking powder	Leavening in baked goods
Disodium phosphate	Anti-caking agent in cereals and pastas; component in cheese making
MSG (monosodium glutamate)	Flavor enhancer
Sodium acid pyrophosphate	Leavener in baked goods
Sodium alginate	Preservative in condiments; additive for smoothness in dairy products, such as chocolate milk and ice cream
Sodium benzoate	Preservative in condiments, sauces, and salad dressings
Sodium hydroxide	Additive to soften and loosen skins of ripe olives and other fruits and vegetables
Sodium nitrate	Curing agent for meats and sausages
Sodium propionate	Additive to inhibit growth of molds in pasteurized cheese and in breads and cakes
Sodium sulfite	Preservative in some dried fruits, such as apricots and plums, and to bleach artificially colored fruits, such as maraschino cherries
Sodium tripolyphosphate	Additive to help retain moisture in shellfish, such as shrimp
Trisodium phosphate	Emulsifier in sauces

Find the Hidden Sodium

Reading nutrition facts panels is truly the only way to find the sneaky, surprising sources of sodium that add up without your realizing it. Thousands of processed foods are sources of this hidden sodium, and many of them don't even taste salty. Common sources of surprising sodium include breads, cereals, and dairy products, as well as add-ons such as condiments, salad dressings, and sauces, which can turn otherwise low-sodium food into sodium traps. Even sweets can be deceptive: on the tongue, the combination of fat, sugar, and sodium creates the taste perception that a cookie is deliciously sweet, when in fact it can be as high in sodium as a salted pretzel. When you start reading and comparing labels, remember that more than 75 percent of the sodium you eat comes from processed food. You might be surprised by just how much sodium the "unsalty" sources contribute to your daily intake. Once you realize that a certain food is likely to be high in sodium, you can rethink how you use that food and decide whether to do without it, reduce it, or replace it with a lower-sodium choice.

Find the Sodium in Unlabeled Foods and at Restaurants

What about foods that aren't packaged and/or don't have a nutrition facts label? Many unprocessed foods—vegetables, fruit, poultry, meat, and seafood—fall into this category. The USDA provides nutrition information for thousands of foods, both processed and unprocessed. Because of all the variables concerning nutritional content that are involved—such as where the foods are grown or raised and how they are handled before they reach the market—the government analyses of foods are typically averages taken from tests of several samples. Although these numbers may not precisely reflect the unlabeled foods you buy, they will give you a good estimate of how much sodium (and other nutrients) a type of food contains.

To find specific nutrition information for products without nutrition facts labels, try these handy resources:

- Part III, "Sodium Sense by Food Type—with Recipes"
- Reliable online sources, such as academic and government websites, including http://ndb.nal.usda.gov/ndb/foods/list
- Food wholesalers and local producers and growers (check with your store manager)
- Pocket nutrition guides in bookstores

Eating out poses challenges, too, since it can be difficult to identify the amount of sodium in restaurant foods. However, most chain restaurants now provide nutrition analyses of their food online and on-site, so it is possible to find out how much sodium is in your favorite menu items and compare dishes to make better choices. You can also ask for information at individual restaurants; if none is available, assume that the dishes are as high in sodium as a similar processed food would be. For example, a typical cheese enchilada combines a flour tortilla, sauce, and, of course, cheese—all of which are high-sodium ingredients—so it's a good bet that any restaurant version will be packed with sodium as well. (Many of the pocket nutrition food guides found in bookstores contain nutrition information on restaurant foods.) Once you become familiar with the typical amounts of sodium in restaurant foods you enjoy, you can apply that knowledge when you're deciding what to order.

Chapter 5, "Target High-Sodium Foods at Home," and Chapter 6, "Identify High-Sodium Foods When Eating Out," explore in more detail where to find the sodium in your pantry and in restaurant kitchens so you can make smart food choices both at home and away from home.

TRACK YOUR CURRENT EATING HABITS

An important part of lowering your sodium intake is finding out how much is in your diet now, and the best way to educate yourself about this is to track your current eating habits. Keeping a detailed log may seem like a lot of trouble at first thought, but the payback is well worth the effort, and you only have to go through the initial process once to see where the sodium comes from. Unless you're writing down exactly what you eat and drink, you probably aren't gauging your sodium intake accurately. Remember, if you are like most other people, you probably are underestimating how much sodium you regularly consume.

Write Down Your Sodium Intake

To get a realistic picture of your sodium intake and heighten your awareness of the food choices you make, keep a log or journal of your eating habits for easy self-monitoring. The act of recording everything you eat and drink for a set period of time makes you more conscious of your actions. This awareness can help you identify your motivations and give you insights into how to change your behavior. At the end of the tracking period, the data you have recorded will give you a snapshot of your typical diet.

To be effective, your food tracker should include *everything* that you consume for at least one week. (Plan to track your sodium intake during an average week that reflects your typical activities and lifestyle.) Record *all* your meals, snacks, and beverages, the salt you add at the table, and even medications you take. Include how much you ate or drank and how much sodium is in each item. Also, think about *why* you chose that particular food or drink. Do you pick up fast food most nights on the way home from work because you are short on time? Do you enjoy a bag of pretzels while watching sports on the weekend because you gravitate toward foods that are crunchy? To record your meals, drinks, snacks, and medications, use any method that works for you—an online list, your smartphone, or an old-fashioned piece of paper. You'll find a blank Daily Sodium Tracker in the Toolkit (page 254) that you can copy and use as a starting point.

Once you've collected an entire week's worth of data, calculate the daily sodium totals, add them up, and divide by 7 to get your average daily sodium intake. When you compare your average intake to 1,500 mg (the American Heart Association recommended daily limit), you'll see how close your result is to the recommendation.

> **SODIUM IN MEDICATIONS** **Many over-the-counter and prescription medications contain sodium in the form of compounds, such as sodium bicarbonate, sodium chloride, and sodium biphosphate. For example, two popular antacid tablets can contain more than 1,000 mg sodium. Other examples include laxatives, antibiotics, and nonsteroidal anti-inflammatory drugs (NSAIDs). Manufacturers are now required to list the sodium content on prescription drug labels, and the FDA has also established labeling rules for nonprescription drugs. Ask your pharmacist for help.**

Take One Step at a Time

Once you know how much sodium is in your diet, assuming that it exceeds 1,500 mg, you can decide how to reduce your intake. The next five chapters of the book offer accessible strategies that should work with your lifestyle.

> **CHECK YOUR BLOOD PRESSURE** **Before you make any sweeping changes, consider visiting your healthcare provider to determine the status of your health, especially your blood pressure. (You can also have your blood pressure checked at a clinic or pharmacy, or with an at-home blood pressure monitor.) Talk to your doctor about which lifestyle modifications will best complement a lower-sodium diet for you.**

Once you've implemented the suggestions in one chapter, take a few weeks to let the new changes become habits. After using one of these strategies for an extended period, say several weeks, go back to tracking your sodium for another week. How much have you been able to reduce your intake? Also, measure your blood pressure again and compare the results with your blood pressure levels from before. Wait until you feel ready—and until your taste buds adjust—before you move on to the next step so the details won't seem overwhelming. Keep in mind that it takes time for your palate to adjust to lower-sodium options and that the benefits of this process are cumulative. However, even the smallest step you take to reduce sodium in your diet is a step toward better heart health.

CHAPTER 4

Start with Small Changes

Owen's Story: *"I travel by plane several times a month for business and was in the habit of ordering a can of Bloody Mary mix when the beverage cart came by. I've got three teenagers now, and I've decided I need to take care of my health for my family. But once I started paying more attention to what I actually ate and drank, I began to notice how some of my 'little' choices really added up. For example, when I saw the nutrition information on the back of the can of that mix, I couldn't believe my eyes. Just 8 ounces contain 1,150 mg of sodium! I was stunned. I had no idea that I was getting so much sodium in that one beverage. Knowing what I know now, I've made the decision to switch to another drink. I don't miss my old standby, and I save myself several thousand milligrams of sodium a month just by making one small change."*

In an ideal world of good health, all of us would eat fresh, unprocessed, or minimally processed foods that are low in sodium. In real life, though, we eat the foods that are readily available to us, especially those that we enjoy and that fit into our lifestyles, budgets, and schedules.

If you are like most other people, among the many decisions you make each day about what to eat, you include lots of processed foods and restaurant fare instead of options that tend to be healthier, including lower-sodium foods. By making better choices *most of the time*, however, you can lower the total amount of sodium in your diet to a healthy level. You don't have to make sweeping all-or-nothing changes to gain control—just start with a few small adjustments in ways that make sense for you and will have the most impact on your sodium intake. Being aware of the sodium in your food choices will also make you mindful of how those choices add up over time.

Rethink. Replace. Reduce. As you begin the transition to a lower-sodium diet, you'll apply these three basic strategies to each step along the way.

SODIUM SHAKEDOWN STRATEGIES

- ✓ Identify the patterns and personal pitfalls that result in added sodium in your diet.
- ✓ Rethink your eating habits and determine which foods you can live without.
- ✓ Replace the highest-sodium items in your diet with lower-sodium alternatives.
- ✓ Reduce your portion size and/or eat high-sodium foods less often.

IDENTIFY YOUR SODIUM SOURCES

Now that you've tracked exactly what you've eaten for a week, as recommended in Chapter 3, your next step is to identify which foods and/or habits pose your biggest sodium threats. (If you haven't started tracking your sodium intake yet, see the Toolkit, Part IV, page 254, for a blank template.) Do you eat out often? Are your portions extra large? Do you eat lots of salty snacks during the day? Don't be tempted to just guess about what you're eating and drinking. Recording and analyzing your food choices for at least one week is an important exercise that will help you understand where the sodium in your diet *actually* comes from, rather than where you *assume* it comes from.

Almost everyone finds one or two—or more—sodium surprises when they look closely at what they're really eating and drinking. Perhaps you don't leave the office for lunch or you get home late from work, so you eat a lot of frozen prepared entrées. For example, a typical frozen chicken entrée with pasta and sauce contains between 1,000 and 1,500 mg of sodium per serving. Are you a busy mom who has to get dinner on the table in a hurry? If so, you may rely on convenience products that are packed with sodium (a serving of a typical boxed ground beef plus noodles dish contains 600 mg). Or maybe you're trying to bump up your veggie intake, so you've decided to drink mixed-vegetable juice every day (1 cup can contain 480 mg). Whatever your unique habits may be, your sodium tracker will reflect them.

Find Your Sodium "Hot" Spots

The average American today eats what is called the Western diet. This type of diet includes a lot of red meat and fatty foods and is high in added salt, sugar, saturated fat, trans fat, and cholesterol. To make matters worse, the Western diet also typically lacks healthier foods, such as vegetables and whole grains, and therefore is low in the nutrients, phytochemicals, and fiber that we need for good health.

Where do you think you fall on the healthy-eating spectrum?

- Do your usual food choices resemble the Western diet more than not?
- Do you try to eat healthy but know that you sometimes fall short of your intentions?
- Do you believe that, for the most part, your diet reflects healthy guidelines?

The unsettling fact is that however health conscious you may or may not be, you are still probably eating too much sodium. Most people know that they could do more to improve their diets in some way, but eating healthy does not guarantee a sodium intake lower than average. In fact, even if you are currently eating a prudent diet that includes lots of nutritious options, you may be unaware of the ways you're letting sodium sabotage your best efforts to stay healthy.

Consider this typical three-day diet sample for an "average" person with an average sodium intake; this could even be you! If you're like this typical person, you start off the day with a reasonably satisfying breakfast. Even so, you often get hungry between meals and keep some snacks on hand for pick-me-ups. You work full time and often grab lunch at quick-casual restaurants or fast-food places during the week. You eat dinner at home most nights, but you tend to use some packaged and/or frozen foods to make dinner preparation quick and easy. One night a week you meet friends for dinner at a favorite pizza place.

On the following pages is a sample sodium shakedown for three days of tracking these "average" food choices. (Items are commercially prepared unless otherwise specified.) The average sodium intake for these three days is more than 4,000 mg. As you review these trackers, think about the following:

- Are you surprised to see how the sodium adds up?
- Do you recognize any of your own typical meal choices?
- Do you see any obvious choices this person can make to easily cut back on the sodium?

DAY 1

FOODS AND BEVERAGES	SERVING SIZE	SODIUM (MG)*
breakfast		
cornflakes with	1 cup	200
fat-free milk	4 oz	50
strawberries	6	0
coffee, black, unsweetened	8 oz	0
	subtotal	**250**
snack		
fat-free yogurt, blueberry	6 oz	**85**
lunch		
fast-food ¼-lb burger with	3-oz patty with bun	470
American cheese	2 slices	430
ketchup	1 tbsp	170
pickles	4 slices	80
french fries	3 oz	350
iced tea, unsweetened	8 oz	0
	subtotal	**1,500**
snack		
pretzels	1 snack pack (1 oz)	**385**
dinner		
homemade beef and broccoli stir-fry with	1 cup	550
soy sauce (added at the table)	1 tbsp	1,000
steamed rice	1 cup	5
iced tea, unsweetened	8 oz	0
	subtotal	**1,555**
	total	3,775

***Sodium values have been rounded to the nearest 5 mg.**

DAY 2

FOODS AND BEVERAGES	SERVING SIZE	SODIUM (MG)*
breakfast		
frozen whole-wheat waffles with	2 4-inch	400
pancake syrup	¼ cup	55
light tub margarine	1 tsp	35
coffee, black, unsweetened	8 oz	0
	subtotal	**490**
snack		
navel orange, medium	1	**0**
lunch		
submarine sandwich of		
whole-grain bread	1 6-inch length	310
turkey breast	2 oz	500
lettuce, tomatoes, onion	1 layer each	0
light mayonnaise	2 tbsp	200
pepperjack cheese	2 slices	160
regular cola	12 oz	50
	subtotal	**1,220**
snack		
baked potato chips	1 snack pack (1 oz)	**200**
dinner		
frozen lasagna with meat sauce with	10-oz container	830
Parmesan cheese (added at the table)	2 tbsp	150
fresh zucchini slices cooked with	¾ cup	0
Italian herbs	½ tsp	0
salt	1/16 tsp	145
garlic bread	1 slice (2-inch)	250
red wine	4 oz	5
ice cream sandwich, fat-free	1	150
	subtotal	**1,530**
	total	3,440

*Sodium values have been rounded to the nearest 5 mg.

DAY 3

FOODS AND BEVERAGES	SERVING SIZE	SODIUM (MG)*
breakfast		
scrambled egg with	1 large	70
salt	1/16 tsp	145
English muffin with	2 halves	200
light tub margarine	1 tsp	35
coffee, black, unsweetened	8 oz	0
	subtotal	**450**
snack		
protein bar	1 oz	**110**
lunch		
"healthy" salad bar selections of		
mixed salad greens and spinach	3 cups	65
mushrooms	1/8 cup	0
artichoke hearts, marinated	1/4 cup	210
bacon bits	2 tbsp	260
tuna salad	1/4 cup	375
croutons	1/4 cup	390
ranch dressing	1/4 cup	495
corn bread mini muffin	1	75
iced tea, unsweetened	12 oz	0
	subtotal	**1,870**
snack		
mini wheat crackers	16 pieces	**310**
dinner		
deep-dish pepperoni pizza	2 slices of 14-inch pie	2,240
beer	12 oz	10
	subtotal	**2,250**
	total	4,990

***Sodium values have been rounded to the nearest 5 mg.**

When compared to the recommended limit of 1,500 mg of sodium a day, an intake of more than 4,000 mg of sodium seems extreme. Nevertheless, for the thousands of average Americans who rely on processed foods and fast-food meals every day, it is a reality. If you're one of them, keeping an account of what you are eating will dramatically illustrate where your "sodium hot spots" are and where you can make adjustments. No matter where your sodium intake falls at the moment, your own tracker will allow you to see what you're doing right, as well as how you can improve.

For example, a trip to the salad bar may seem like a healthy alternative to sandwiches and burgers, but as you can see from the lunchtime sodium values for Day 3, it all depends on what you choose to put on your plate. Cooking at home can be a great way to control your eating habits, but if you serve your entrée with an add-on that contains two-thirds of a day's worth of sodium—as our "average" person did for dinner on Day 1—you've defeated your purpose.

Focus on Your High-Sodium Items

After you have tracked your sodium intake for a week, review and assess the information that you collected. Look for the entries that represent the highest percentage of your sodium intake and make a chart of the top items, starting with the one that has the highest sodium content. Start with the totals, but be sure to break down combination foods, such as sandwiches, so you can see which ingredients are the worst offenders. Having a list of these will help you find the high-impact changes that will give you the most reduction in sodium with the least effort.

Here's how the high-sodium items in the three-day sample would break down:

TOP HIGH-SODIUM MEALS	TOTAL SODIUM (MG)*
deep-dish pepperoni pizza	2,240
salad bar	1,870
homemade beef and broccoli stir-fry including rice and soy sauce added at the table	1,555
fast-food ¼-lb burger with cheese, ketchup, and pickles and a side of french fries	1,500
frozen lasagna dinner including zucchini and bread	1,375
6-inch submarine sandwich	1,170

***Sodium values have been rounded to the nearest 5 mg.**

With everything laid out on paper, it's easy to see where the biggest problems are. Two of these high-sodium meals contain at least two-thirds of one day's total sodium allowance. Two others contain an *entire* day's worth, and the two highest-sodium offenders contain *more than* the recommended daily limit of 1,500 mg—in just one meal. As you'll learn on the following pages, finding ways to replace, reduce, or do without just a few of the problem items could make a difference of almost 1,000 mg of sodium per day!

Identify Patterns and Pitfalls

Your weeklong sodium tracker will also provide a record of the patterns that recur in your eating habits and preferences. What crops up every other day or meal? Are your breakfasts, lunches, or snacks the same every day? Do you have a few favorites that you usually order when you eat out? Perhaps you always grab a snack pack of pretzels when you're bored (500 mg), love a crisp dill pickle with your sandwich (an extra 660 mg), or order fajitas on Fridays (4,800 mg). This is the information you need to know so *you can make changes now for the quickest impact.*

Look at your own tracker to identify these patterns. Becoming aware of the reasons you choose one thing instead of another allows you to see exactly how routines and seemingly random choices define your eating habits. Can you identify the circumstances that lead you to make the choices you do? Sometimes it's environment (at work, you eat in the cafeteria and have no access to lower-sodium options); other times, it's scheduling (you have no time to cook between getting home and getting to the kids' activities).

Personal preferences and social situations also play an important role, of course. Maybe you just like the pepperoni pizza at the nearby Italian restaurant and always get it because it's reliable and comforting, and you don't want to think about what to order every time. Whatever reasons lie behind your current eating patterns, identifying them is the first step toward finding lower-sodium alternatives. Then you can decide what you want to change in your circumstances and behaviors and how to go about making those changes.

RETHINK, REPLACE, AND REDUCE

It's time to get to work. Armed with concrete information from your sodium tracker, you've identified the highest-sodium items you ate and have recognized your patterns and pitfalls. Now ask how you can use that information to come up with quick fixes—things you can change easily. Use these three simple strategies to easily knock out some of the sodium in your diet:

- *Rethink* and do without.
- *Replace* with a lower-sodium choice.
- *Reduce* the amount you use or use it less often.

Rethink Your Habits: What Can You Easily Eliminate?

When you review your tracker, if you see high-sodium items that you ate more from habit than from need, ask yourself if you can just do without them. What foods, drinks, or condiments wouldn't you miss? For example, that dill pickle may seem like the perfect companion for your sandwich because it automatically comes with the lunch you order at the deli. Do you enjoy eating the pickle, or do you eat it because it's there? Is it really worth the 660 mg of sodium it adds? If a high-sodium food, such as the pickle, is not a major component of your meal and does not contribute to the nutritional balance of your diet, consider dropping it from your meal.

Using the three-day tracker examples, if you can eliminate even a few add-ons to your meals, you will substantially cut back on your sodium intake.

RETHINK

DO WITHOUT THESE . . .	TO SAVE THIS MUCH SODIUM (MG)* PER SERVING
on stir-fry:	
1 tbsp soy sauce (added at the table)	1,000
on fast-food burger:	
2 slices American cheese	430
1 tbsp ketchup	170
from salad bar selections:	
2 tbsp bacon bits	260
total sodium savings	1,860

***Sodium values have been rounded to the nearest 5 mg.**

Consider the many high-sodium add-ons that you are likely to encounter, especially at restaurants: shredded cheese and croutons at the salad bar, soy sauce for sushi or stir-fries, even the salt on a margarita glass. When you rethink the "cost" of so many side sources of sodium, you may find it easier than you expected simply to do without them. If you're not ready to go cold turkey, however, you can also start by indulging less often.

Replace the High with the Healthy: What Can You Easily Substitute?

Once you've studied your tracker and identified which foods and beverages are the highest in sodium, you can begin to replace them with lower-sodium choices, such as switching from a high-sodium brand of bread to a lower one, choosing a different type of cereal, or ordering a different menu item when eating out. When you make smart substitutions on a regular basis, even a few swaps can save you a substantial amount of sodium.

REPLACE

REPLACE THIS MEAL OR ADD-ON . . .	SODIUM (MG)*	WITH THIS . . .	SODIUM (MG)*	FOR A SAVINGS OF . . .
2 slices deep-dish pepperoni piza	2,240	2 slices vegetable pizza, regular crust	1,120	**1,120**
10-oz container frozen lasagna	830	1 serving homemade lasagna, such as *Family Night Lasagna* (page 188), stored in freezer	490	**340**
1 cup cornflakes	200	1 cup shredded wheat minis	0	**200**
on sub sandwich: 2 tbsp light mayonnaise	200	1 tbsp oil and vinegar	0	**200**
			total sodium savings	**1,860**

***Sodium values have been rounded to the nearest 5 mg.**

Make small changes in your eating pattern to eliminate the biggest sources of sodium. This strategy works especially well if your tracker shows that you tend to stick to predictable routines that can be easily reoriented. For more ideas, see "Sodium-Savvy Substitutions" in the Toolkit (Part IV, page 256).

Reduce the Portion Size: What Can You Easily Cut Back On?

Eating less is a good way to reduce your sodium intake without needing to think too much or keep records of what you eat. By cutting back on the amount of food you consume, you automatically cut out a proportional amount of sodium. For example, eating half the usual amount of the high-sodium sides and snacks you've identified allows you to continue to enjoy those foods *and* reduce sodium at the same time. For foods that are add-ons, try eating them half as often as you normally would or put half as much on your plate. As a bonus, if you need to lose weight, this reduced-portion approach can help you transition to a way of eating that is lower in both sodium and calories.

REDUCE

REPLACE THIS MEAL OR ADD-ON . . .	SODIUM (MG)*	WITH THIS . . .	SODIUM (MG)*	FOR A SAVINGS OF . . .
2 slices deep-dish pepperoni pizza	2,240	1 slice	1,120	**1,120**
fast-food ¼-lb burger with cheese, ketchup, and pickles	1,150	fast-food "junior" burger with cheese, ketchup, and pickles	610	**540**
10-oz container frozen lasagna	830	7-oz container frozen lasagna	650	**180**
on stir-fry:				
1 tbsp soy sauce	1,000	1 tsp	335	**665**
from salad bar:				
¼ cup tuna salad	375	2 tbsp	185	**185**
¼ cup ranch dressing	495	2 tbsp	245	**245**
on sub sandwich:				
2 tbsp light mayonnaise	200	1 tbsp	100	**100**
2 slices pepperjack cheese	160	1 slice	80	**80**
			total sodium savings	3,115

*Sodium values have been rounded to the nearest 5 mg.

Using the high-sodium foods from the sample tracker on pages 49–51, you can quickly see how the numbers add up to reduce sodium intake when portions are reduced.

This approach allows you to reduce the amount of high-sodium food you eat in any situation, which makes it a good strategy for times when you aren't in control of the foods you have to choose from, such as when you are traveling, dining out, or at a dinner party. Take the time to learn about the foods and beverages you'll encounter that are most likely to be high in sodium, such as bread, cold cuts, cheese, burgers, pizza, and snacks. The more you know, the more you will be able to accurately gauge what to eat freely and what to eat in smaller portions.

CHANGE OLD HABITS INTO NEW BEHAVIORS

To start changing your eating habits right now, use the strategies of rethink, replace, and reduce with the information you collected in Chapter 3 to create your own start-up action plan. Choose the high-sodium foods from your tracker you want to tackle first, then decide which strategy will bring you the greatest sodium savings. Consider how to put your sodium-savings plan into action and commit to follow through on the choices you make. Whatever small changes you start with at the beginning, be sure they are realistic and make sense for your current lifestyle.

Start Simple

In the sample savings plan on the next page, our "average" person uses rethink, replace, and reduce to find the easiest ways to save the most sodium. If this scenario reflects your own typical eating habits, by making the changes with the most impact, you could reduce the sodium in these meals by almost half! Even if you acted on only a few of these changes, you could make a substantial difference in your total sodium intake.

This sample plan is based on the choices of a fictitious person, a composite of "average" behaviors. Using the same technique of analyzing your eating patterns, you can reduce the sodium in your diet as effectively in reality as presented here in theory.

RETHINK, REPLACE, REDUCE: 3-DAY SAMPLE SODIUM SAVINGS

ORIGINAL TOP-HIGHEST FOODS (HIGHEST TO LOWEST)	SODIUM (MG)*	TAKE THIS ACTION . . .	FOR A SAVINGS OF . . .
2 slices deep-dish pepperoni pizza	2,240	REPLACE: Choose 2 slices regular-crust vegetable pizza	**1,120**
from the salad bar:			
2 tbsp bacon bits	260	RETHINK: Do without	**260**
¼ cup tuna salad	375	REDUCE: Choose 2 tbsp	**185**
¼ cup ranch dressing	495	REDUCE: Choose 2 tbsp	**245**
on stir-fry:			
1 tbsp soy sauce (added at the table)	1,000	RETHINK: Do without	**1,000**
10-oz container frozen lasagna	830	REPLACE: Make homemade version, such as *Family Night Lasagna* (page 188)	**340**
on fast-food burger:			
2 slices American cheese	430	RETHINK: Do without	**430**
1 tbsp ketchup	170	REDUCE: Choose 1 tsp	**55**
on sub sandwich:			
2 tbsp light mayonnaise	200	REPLACE: Choose oil and vinegar	**200**
2 slices pepperjack cheese	160	REDUCE: Choose 1 slice	**80**
3-day totals	6,160		3,915

***Sodium values have been rounded to the nearest 5 mg.**

Graduate Slowly, Step-by-Step

Remember that once you do the basic legwork to become sodium-savvy, cutting back gradually will become easier. It is helpful to create a personal sodium reference tool—a smartphone app such as Good Food–Bad Food and MyFitnessPal or a small notebook and pencil—and enter the names and sodium counts of the foods and beverages you are likely to eat or drink often. Once you determine the sodium content of your favorite ravioli, for example, you'll always have that number on record for future tracking and to gauge how that food fits into your sodium budget on any given day. When you go food shopping, take your reference with you and record new entries to keep expanding your base of knowledge. Also, keep a record of lower-sodium restaurant alternatives so that when you're eating out, you'll remember what to order.

Another way to put an easy fix to work is by stair-stepping from a really high-sodium item to one that's somewhat lower sodium, then to a low- or even no-sodium alternative. If, like so many people, your regular diet includes the popular foods and drinks that make up such a big part of the American diet, you can gradually transition from the regular option to a better one—and finally to the best.

The chart below gives you some ideas on how to start.

REGULAR OPTION	BETTER OPTION	BEST OPTION
fast-food crispy fried chicken breast	fast-food chicken nuggets, 6 pieces	grilled chicken breast, plain
fast-food fish sandwich	homemade tuna fish sandwich	grilled tuna, 3 oz cooked
smoked ham, 3 oz	turkey bacon, 4 slices	grilled pork chop, 3 oz
potato salad, deli-style, ½ cup	mashed potatoes, ½ cup	baked potato with chives
salted peanuts, ¼ cup	peanut butter, low-sodium, 1 tbsp	unsalted peanuts, ¼ cup
salsa, restaurant-style, ¼ cup	"fresh" style salsa, ¼ cup	homemade salsa, ¼ cup

Quick fixes can give you quick solutions, but there are several other strategies for you to explore that will lead to even greater sodium savings. Do you know what foods in your pantry, fridge, and freezer contribute most to your sodium intake? To find out, check out Chapter 5, "Target High-Sodium Foods at Home." Do you eat out frequently or bring home take-out? If so, see the strategies that Chapter 6, "Identify High-Sodium Foods When Eating Out," can offer you. Do you like to cook? If so, the strategies in Chapter 8, "Plan Ahead with Lower-Sodium Menus," and the recipes in Part III will best complement your lifestyle. No matter which strategies you choose to adopt a lower-sodium lifestyle, be sure to refer also to Chapter 7, "Stay Focused on Eating Well," and Chapter 9, "Healthy Sodium for Life," for recommendations on how to establish healthy eating habits and enjoy an overall healthy lifestyle.

CHAPTER 5

Target High-Sodium Foods at Home

Christy's Story: *"My husband and I are both pretty health conscious. We shop for organic and local foods, avoid fast food, and cook at home for the family. I thought we were doing a good job, until I took a long, hard look at the products I relied on most of the time. I certainly didn't realize how much sodium we were eating! I figured that our intake would be way under the national average [3,400 mg sodium a day], but I was so wrong. When I started adding up the sodium that was sitting on my pantry shelves and in my refrigerator and freezer, I was astounded. I had no idea how much sodium was in some of my go-to staples like tomato sauce, garlic salt, and mustard, not to mention all those boxes of rice pilaf! Since that wake-up call, I'm a much more careful shopper. Now I always check the nutrition facts panel for sodium. I still love to try new foods, and I really like the convenience of packaged side dishes, but I am much smarter about how often I use them and how much I serve."*

Every household has its own unique "food culture." The food culture in your family affects the way you think about food and eating, as well as the food-related decisions you make. If you are an experienced cook with three children, your needs will be very different from those of a young single guy who doesn't like to cook, and of course, the food in the two kitchens will reflect these differences. Yet, despite their very disparate cooking habits and food preferences, these two people will probably find they have one thing in common: an excess of sodium in their kitchens.

Almost everyone faces the same challenges when it comes to trying to keep sodium low, and chances are you do, too. Take a moment to think about your food culture and how it affects your eating habits and how you shop for food. For example, you may believe that because you're cooking at home, you have your sodium under control, but if you use a lot of packaged and processed foods, you may be surprised to see how much they contribute to your family's sodium intake. Next, get ready to do a "sodium spring cleaning" in your kitchen to identify the sodium-filled foods and beverages that you can rethink, replace, or reduce.

SODIUM SHAKEDOWN STRATEGIES

- ✓ Review your pantry, refrigerator, and freezer to find the high-sodium foods and beverages.
- ✓ Identify the patterns and habits that reinforce your use of high-sodium foods.
- ✓ Rethink your choices to find the foods you can live without.
- ✓ Replace the highest-sodium items in your kitchen with lower-sodium or sodium-free alternatives.
- ✓ Reduce portions of high-sodium products and/or how often you use them to reduce your overall sodium intake.
- ✓ Repeat a kitchen sodium sweep after a few weeks.

ASSESS YOUR SODIUM SOURCES IN YOUR KITCHEN

As soon as you're ready to tackle the job of reducing the sodium in your kitchen, take an inventory of all your foods and beverages. Do a methodical, shelf-by-shelf search of all your pantry items, checking the nutrition facts panels on them and writing down how much sodium is in a serving of each item. Make a note of any foods that are not labeled so you can look them up separately; the charts in Part III, "Sodium Sense by Food Type—with Recipes," are handy starting points for this information. When you've finished with the pantry, move on to the refrigerator, then the freezer. As you document the sodium in each food, your base of knowledge will expand, and you'll quickly be able to see which items are relatively high and which are low.

The more thorough you are, the better overview you'll have of the sources of sodium in your kitchen. Putting in a little effort now will provide a healthy payback in the long run; and as a bonus, once you've recorded sodium levels for the things you buy regularly, you can just jot down any additional information for new products as you buy them. Many of the items in your kitchen are staples that you use again and again, such as the canned broth you use to make soup and the sauces you use often because your family loves them on pasta. These go-to foods form the basis of your personal food culture, so they are the obvious place for you to start making healthy changes.

While it's natural to focus on finding the items that are highest in sodium, don't be tempted to ignore the foods that might seem insignificant. How often you eat something matters, too, and very often, it's the small amounts of condiments, dressings, and sauces that can rack up sodium surprisingly fast. Whether it's tomato sauce, ketchup, or curry paste, when you add a little bit here and a little bit there, before you know it, you've added thousands of milligrams of sodium to your diet.

DURING YOUR SODIUM SWEEP, LOOK FOR THESE COMMON SOURCES OF SODIUM:

In the pantry

- Packaged foods that include added salt (by itself or in the form of seasoning or flavorings), such as rice-based dishes, pasta-based dishes, and sauce mixes
- Canned foods that contain added salt or sauce, such as beans, vegetables (including tomato products), soups, and tuna
- Cereals, crackers, chips, and breads
- Baking mixes
- Baked goods
- Condiments and sauces

In the spice rack

- Seasoning blends
- Flavored salts, such as garlic salt and onion salt

In the fridge

- Dairy products, such as cheese, sour cream, and milk
- Salad dressings, condiments, and spreads
- Deli meats and hot dogs
- Beverages, such as sport drinks and mixers

In the freezer

- Poultry, meat, and seafood
- Vegetable combinations with sauces
- Prepared entrées, sides, and breakfast foods
- Fast-food entrées, such as pizza, chicken nuggets, and burritos

In the medicine cabinet

- Prescription and over-the-counter drugs, such as antacids and many antibiotics

Study a Sample Sodium Sweep

The chart below and continued through page 66 shows the results of a sodium sweep through the pantry, refrigerator, and freezer of Christy, the stay-at-home mom you met in Chapter 3. Christy shops several times a week because she prefers fresh vegetables, fruit, and seafood, but she also likes to keep frozen and canned staples on hand so she can cook a meal quickly without having to run to the store first. These entries reflect what Christy finds in her kitchen when she checks the sodium in her typical food choices, as well as how often she uses a particular item. (For the purposes of this example, *often* is defined as once a week or more, *occasionally* as less than once a week but at least twice a month, and *rarely* as once a month or less.)

IN STAY-AT-HOME MOM CHRISTY'S KITCHEN

PANTRY	SODIUM PER SERVING (MG)*	FREQUENCY OF USE
broths, canned		
beef, fat-free	890 per 1 cup	often
chicken, low-fat	860 per 1 cup	often
soups, canned		
chicken noodle, condensed	890 per 1 cup prepared	often
cream of mushroom, condensed	830 per ½ cup condensed	occasionally
vegetables, canned		
corn, organic	360 per ½ cup	occasionally
green peas	380 per ½ cup	occasionally
green beans, organic	380 per ½ cup	often
artichoke quarters	210 per 4 pieces	rarely
beans, canned		
black	460 per ½ cup	often
chickpeas	440 per ½ cup	occasionally
kidney	335 per ½ cup	often
pinto	360 per ½ cup	rarely
cannellini	390 per ½ cup	rarely
tomato products, canned		
diced tomatoes, "100% natural"	310 per ½ cup	often
tomato sauce, "100% natural"	410 per ¼ cup	often
tomato paste	105 per 2 tbsp	rarely
spaghetti sauces, various flavors	375 to 520 per ½ cup	often

***Sodium values have been rounded to the nearest 5 mg.**

CONTINUED

PANTRY	SODIUM PER SERVING (MG)*	FREQUENCY OF USE
sauces, seasonings, and condiments		
salsa	500 per ¼ cup	often
hoisin sauce	230 per 1 tbsp	occasionally
tartar sauce	125 per 1 tbsp	occasionally
mustard, yellow	165 per 1 tbsp	occasionally
mustard, Dijon	360 per 1 tbsp	often
mayonnaise, real	90 per 1 tbsp	often
Worcestershire sauce	165 per 1 tbsp	occasionally
Louisiana hot sauce	240 per 1 tsp	rarely
ketchup	170 per 1 tbsp	often
cocktail sauce	760 per ¼ cup	occasionally
soy sauce	1,000 per 1 tbsp	often
chili powder	20 per ½ tsp	often
garlic salt	240 per ¼ tsp	often
pasta, rice, and grains		
pasta	0 per 2 oz	often
brown rice, regular	0 per ½ cup cooked	often
long-grain and wild rice mix, seasoned	390 per ½ cup cooked	rarely
brown rice pilaf mix, organic	530 per ½ cup cooked	often
Thai-style noodle mix	800 per ⅔ cup cooked	rarely
macaroni and cheese mix, organic	900 per 1 cup cooked	occasionally
skillet Stroganoff mix	750 per 1 cup cooked	occasionally
cereals		
whole-grain clusters	290 per 1 cup	often
oatmeal	0 per ¾ cup	occasionally
oat rings	160 per 1 cup	often
shredded wheat minis	0 per 1¼ cup	often
crackers, chips, and snacks		
whole-wheat crackers, organic	225 per 6 crackers	often
rye crispbreads	70 per 2 slices	occasionally
graham crackers	180 per 8 pieces	rarely
tortilla chips	150 per 1 oz	often
potato chips with sea salt	160 per 1 oz	often
pretzels, fat-free, salted	485 per 2 large	often
popcorn, light microwave	220 per 1 oz popped	often

***Sodium values have been rounded to the nearest 5 mg.**

PANTRY	SODIUM PER SERVING (MG)*	FREQUENCY OF USE
baking products		
baking soda	155 per ⅛ tsp	occasionally
cornstarch	0 per 1 tbsp	often
gelatin, plain	15 per 1 envelope	rarely
molasses, dark	20 per 1 tbsp	rarely
condensed milk	45 per 2 tbsp	rarely
breads		
whole wheat	160 per 1 slice	occasionally
rye	200 per 1 slice	often
English muffin	200 per muffin	often
pizza crust, packaged	350 per ⅙ of crust	occasionally
tuna, canned, albacore	315 per 3 oz	often
apple juice, unsweetened	35 per 8 oz	often
green tea with ginseng, bottled	20 per 8 oz	often
olives, green	280 per 6 pieces	rarely
peanut butter, chunky regular	130 per 2 tbsp	often
pudding mix, instant sugar-free	415 per ½-cup serving	often

REFRIGERATOR	SODIUM PER SERVING (MG)*	FREQUENCY OF USE
milk, fat-free	105 per 1 cup	every day
cheeses		
Vermont Cheddar	175 per 1 oz	often
Parmesan	75 per 1 tbsp	often
Swiss	55 per 1 oz	often
yogurt, fat-free	125 per 6 oz	often
sour cream, low-fat	20 per 2 tbsp	rarely
deli ham, honey-baked, 97% fat-free	690 per 2 oz	often
deli turkey breast, fat-free	500 per 2 oz	often

***Sodium values have been rounded to the nearest 5 mg.**

CONTINUED

FREEZER	SODIUM PER SERVING (MG)*	FREQUENCY OF USE
frozen, packaged		
Italian meatballs	460 per 6 meatballs	often
Indian entrée (chicken biryani; 1 serving per container)	1,080 per serving	occasionally
Chinese entrée (shrimp in garlic sauce; 2 servings per container)	1,350 per serving	often
soy burgers	380 per 1 burger	rarely
chicken breasts, cooked	130 per 3 oz	often
shrimp, large (31–40 count)	805 per 3 oz	occasionally
frozen, unpackaged/unlabeled		
chicken breasts, raw	80 per 4 oz	often
tilapia, raw	60 per 4 oz	occasionally
sirloin steak, raw	60 per 4 oz	occasionally
ground beef, 95% lean, raw	100 per 4 oz	often
pork chops, raw	60 per 4 oz	occasionally

***Sodium values have been rounded to the nearest 5 mg.**

Identify Your High-Sodium, High-Frequency Items

By doing the legwork (even if it seems tedious, it will be worth it!) to identify the highest-sodium foods in your kitchen, you are educating yourself so you can decide the best course of action to reduce sodium. Go over the results of your sodium sweep, highlighting the often or occasionally used items that contain more than about 300 mg of sodium per serving. In fact, because frequency of use has such an impact on the total amount of sodium consumed, the best way to show the true impact of each item on your overall sodium intake is to calculate a monthly average for the items you use often (once a week or more).

Using the results from the sample inventory, the chart on pages 67–68 shows the top offenders in Christy's kitchen, with a monthly average of total sodium. To create a similar chart of your own, pull out each high-sodium item you've highlighted and estimate how many servings you use each week. Multiply the weekly sodium in each item by 4 to see about how much sodium that food or beverage contributes to your diet over a month's time.

TOP HIGH-SODIUM ITEMS IN CHRISTY'S KITCHEN

	SODIUM PER SERVING (MG)*	HOW OFTEN USED (ESTIMATE)	MONTHLY AVERAGE SODIUM (MG)*
soy sauce	1,000 per 1 tbsp	2 x per week	8,000
chicken noodle soup, condensed	890 per 1 cup prepared	2 x per week	7,120
chicken broth, low-fat	860 per 1 cup	2 x per week	6,880
deli ham, honey-baked, 97% fat-free	690 per 2 oz	2 x per week	5,520
frozen Chinese entrée (shrimp in garlic sauce; 2 servings per container)	1,350 per serving	1 x per week	5,400
brown rice pilaf mix, organic	530 per ½ cup cooked	2 x per week	4,240
salsa	500 per ¼ cup	2 x per week	4,000
pretzels, fat-free, salted	485 per 2 large	2 x per week	3,880
garlic salt	240 per ¼ tsp	4 x per week	3,840
spaghetti sauces, various flavors	average 450 per ½ cup	2 x per week	3,600
beef broth, fat-free	890 per 1 cup	1 x per week	3,560
whole-grain cluster cereal	290 per 1 cup	3 x per week	3,480
tomato sauce	410 per ¼ cup	2 x per week	3,280
mustard, Dijon	360 per 1 tbsp	2 x per week	2,880
whole-wheat crackers, organic	225 per 6 crackers	3 x per week	2,700
diced tomatoes	310 per ½ cup	2 x per week	2,480
frozen Indian entrée (chicken biryani)	1,080 per serving	2 x per month	2,160
ketchup	170 per 1 tbsp	3 x per week	2,040
black beans, canned	460 per ½ cup	1 x per week	1,840

***Sodium values have been rounded to the nearest 5 mg.**

CONTINUED

	SODIUM PER SERVING (MG)*	HOW OFTEN USED (ESTIMATE)	MONTHLY AVERAGE SODIUM (MG)*
Italian meatballs	460 per 6 meatballs	1 x per week	1,840
macaroni and cheese mix, organic	900 per 1 cup cooked	2 x per month	1,800
popcorn, light microwave	220 per 1 oz popped	2 x per week	1,760
instant sugar-free pudding mix	415 per ½-cup serving	1 x per week	1,660
cream of mushroom soup, condensed	830 per ½ cup condensed	2 x per month	1,660
frozen shrimp, large (31–40 count)	805 per 3 oz	2 x per month	1,610
rye bread	200 per 1 slice	2 x per week	1,600
green beans, canned, organic	380 per ½ cup	1 x per week	1,520
cocktail sauce	760 per ¼ cup	2 x per month	1,520
skillet Stroganoff mix	750 per 1 cup cooked	2 x per month	1,500
kidney beans, canned	335 per ½ cup	1 x per week	1,340
tuna, canned, albacore	315 per 3 oz	1 x per week	1,260
tortilla chips	150 per 1 oz	2 x per week	1,200
chickpeas, canned	440 per ½ cup	2 x per month	880

***Sodium values have been rounded to the nearest 5 mg.**

Of course, your own food culture and preferences will dictate the entries in your chart, and many of the examples given will differ from what sits on your pantry shelves and in your refrigerator and freezer. However, the process of analyzing each item to understand its part in your overall sodium intake doesn't change from home to home. For every high-sodium item that you bring into your kitchen, especially those you use most often, it's time to decide on a specific action that will result in your making a lower-sodium choice in the grocery store.

SHOPPING FOR OPTIONS

Look for comparable products for each of your high-sodium items, checking the nutrition facts panels for the serving size as well as the sodium content. If you find several viable options for a certain item, such as the various flavors of spaghetti sauce, write down the specifics of each. First buy the one that most appeals to you. If you try it and find that the brand or flavor doesn't suit your needs after all, try another. Just don't keep buying the same high-sodium product out of habit. For example, when shopping for pasta sauces, you might compare the sodium values for the four varieties below.

Vodka-Style Pasta Sauce

Nutrition Facts	
Serving Size ½ cup	
Servings Per Container About 5	
Amount Per Serving	
Calories 150	Calories from Fat 80
	% Daily Value*
Total Fat 9g	14%
Saturated Fat 4.5g	23%
Trans Fat 0g	0%
Cholesterol 25mg	8%
Sodium 730mg	30%

Five-Cheese Pasta Sauce

Nutrition Facts	
Serving Size ½ cup	
Servings Per Container About 5	
Amount Per Serving	
Calories 100	Calories from Fat 25
	% Daily Value*
Total Fat 3g	5%
Saturated Fat 1g	5%
Trans Fat 0g	0%
Cholesterol 5mg	0%
Sodium 670mg	28%

Tomato and Basil Pasta Sauce

Nutrition Facts	
Serving Size ½ cup	
Servings Per Container About 5	
Amount Per Serving	
Calories 80	Calories from Fat 20
	% Daily Value*
Total Fat 2g	3%
Saturated Fat 0g	0%
Trans Fat 0g	0%
Cholesterol 0mg	0%
Sodium 520mg	22%

Lower-Sodium Marinara Sauce

Nutrition Facts	
Serving Size ½ cup	
Servings Per Container About 5	
Amount Per Serving	
Calories 70	Calories from Fat 30
	% Daily Value*
Total Fat 3g	5%
Saturated Fat 0g	0%
Trans Fat 0g	0%
Cholesterol 0mg	0%
Sodium 250mg	11%

Humans are creatures of habit, and food shopping is a good example of that truism. Without even thinking about it, most of us tend to buy the same types of food, the same brands, year after year. Perhaps your mother used a certain kind of bread, so you do, too, or you always keep a special brand of cereal in the pantry because your husband likes it. Whatever your routine, you may be bringing home more sodium than you need, just out of habit. Compare the sodium values for the four varieties of canned tomatoes below. Notice the difference in sodium between the no-salt-added variety and the three other types.

Organic Diced Tomatoes

Nutrition Facts	
Serving Size ½ cup	
Servings Per Container About 3	
Amount Per Serving	
Calories 25	Calories from Fat 0
	% Daily Value*
Total Fat 0g	0%
Saturated Fat 0g	0%
Trans Fat 0g	0%
Cholesterol 0mg	0%
Sodium 290mg	12%

"100% Natural" Diced Tomatoes

Nutrition Facts	
Serving Size ½ cup	
Servings Per Container About 3.5	
Amount Per Serving	
Calories 30	Calories from Fat 0
	% Daily Value*
Total Fat 0g	0%
Saturated Fat 0g	0%
Trans Fat 0g	0%
Cholesterol 0mg	0%
Sodium 300mg	12%

Imported Diced Tomatoes

Nutrition Facts	
Serving Size ½ cup	
Servings Per Container About 6	
Amount Per Serving	
Calories 25	Calories from Fat 0
	% Daily Value*
Total Fat 0g	0%
Saturated Fat 0g	0%
Trans Fat 0g	0%
Cholesterol 0mg	0%
Sodium 220mg	9%

No-Salt-Added Diced Tomatoes

Nutrition Facts	
Serving Size ½ cup	
Servings Per Container About 3.5	
Amount Per Serving	
Calories 25	Calories from Fat 0
	% Daily Value*
Total Fat 0g	0%
Saturated Fat 0g	0%
Trans Fat 0g	0%
Cholesterol 0mg	0%
Sodium 50mg	2%

Follow the same procedure with all products that are available in a range of sodium levels. Pay special attention to those you use often, such as canned tomatoes and chicken broth, because the differences can really add up.

Familiarizing yourself with the levels of sodium in different brands will also pay off when you're ready to take another step to further reduce your sodium intake. If you know there are even lower sodium options available, you can transition down gradually to the next-lowest amount when you are ready.

Chicken Broth

Nutrition Facts	
Serving Size 1 cup	
Servings Per Container About 4	
Amount Per Serving	
Calories 10	Calories from Fat 0
	% Daily Value*
Total Fat 0.5g	1%
Saturated Fat 0g	0%
Trans Fat 0g	0%
Cholesterol 5mg	2%
Sodium 860mg	36%

33% Reduced-Sodium Chicken Broth

Nutrition Facts	
Serving Size 1 cup	
Servings Per Container About 4	
Amount Per Serving	
Calories 15	Calories from Fat 0
	% Daily Value*
Total Fat 0g	0%
Saturated Fat 0g	0%
Trans Fat 0g	0%
Cholesterol 0	0%
Sodium 570mg	24%

Low-Sodium Chicken Broth

Nutrition Facts	
Serving Size ½ cup	
Servings Per Container About 2	
Amount Per Serving	
Calories 5	Calories from Fat 0
	% Daily Value*
Total Fat 0g	0%
Saturated Fat 0g	0%
Trans Fat 0g	0%
Cholesterol 0mg	0%
Sodium 140mg	6%

Also, remember to compare commercial brands with homemade options, such as Mamma Mia Marinara on page 215, at 16 mg per ½ cup, or Chicken Broth on page 177 at 37 mg per 1 cup. If you find that you absolutely cannot live without an old standby, try using less than your usual amount when you can; you'll automatically be cutting back on your sodium intake.

To change your routine and cut back on sodium at home, record the items that top your personal list of high-sodium offenders. Use the Product Comparison Tracker template in the Toolkit (Part IV, page 259) or create a chart of your own, leaving space to jot down notes as you shop. With this information in hand, you're ready to compare options and look for better choices. The idea is to gain perspective on the choices available at local stores so you can decide which will be the best for you at this stage of your sodium transition. As you get accustomed to using lower-sodium options, you can continue to stair-step down.

When you go shopping, plan to allow enough time to do some in-depth research. As you progress through the grocery store, decide how you want to deal with each item on your chart:

- *Rethink* and do without.
- *Replace* with a lower-sodium choice.
- *Reduce* the amount you use or use it less often.

Understand Labels, Claims, and Icons

For every category of food, you will find an assortment of front-of-package labeling, but all manufacturers must comply with the same rules established by the U.S. government. (See "Know the Sodium Specifics" on page 40 for the details of what the different wordings mean.) For example, a "no salt added" or "unsalted" claim on the label means that no sodium was added during processing; however, it does not mean that the food is sodium free. It's always better to compare the actual sodium value on the nutrition facts panel rather than to rely on labeling terms.

Likewise, terms such as "natural" and "organic" do not mean that a food is also low in sodium. In fact, some of the manufactured products that are advertised as being healthier can actually be higher in sodium than their "regular" counterparts, as the following examples illustrate.

Regular Ketchup

Nutrition Facts	
Serving Size 1 Tb Servings Per Container About 33	
Amount Per Serving	
Calories 20	Calories from Fat 0
	% Daily Value*
Total Fat 0g	0%
Saturated Fat 0g	0%
Trans Fat 0g	0%
Cholesterol 0mg	0%
Sodium 160mg	7%

No-Salt-Added Ketchup

Nutrition Facts	
Serving Size 1 Tb Servings Per Container About 33	
Amount Per Serving	
Calories 25	Calories from Fat 0
	% Daily Value*
Total Fat 0g	0%
Saturated Fat 0g	0%
Trans Fat 0g	0%
Cholesterol 0mg	0%
Sodium 5mg	1%

Organic Ketchup

Nutrition Facts

Serving Size 1 Tb
Servings Per Container About 33

Amount Per Serving	
Calories 20	Calories from Fat 0
	% Daily Value*
Total Fat 0g	0%
Saturated Fat 0g	0%
Trans Fat 0g	0%
Cholesterol 0mg	0%
Sodium 210mg	9%

Several organizations, including the American Heart Association, are working to make it easy to decipher the information on food packaging. Many have developed icon systems to help you make decisions when you shop, and some grocery stores have introduced their own on-shelf labeling programs. When you see a front-of-package icon or wording that signals a health claim, you should still evaluate the information on the nutrition facts panel and the ingredient list before you make your selection. However, when you see a product with the American Heart Association's red-and-white Heart-Check Mark on the label, you can be sure that the product meets the association's limits for total fat, saturated fat, trans fat, cholesterol, and sodium. It also must include a minimum level of one of six beneficial nutrients.

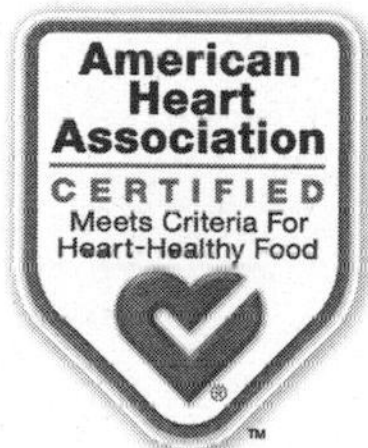

What About Unprocessed Foods?

Comparing labels on processed foods takes a lot of the guesswork out of sodium-smart shopping, but what about the foods that are sold in their natural state, without nutrition information? Although you may assume that these foods contain only naturally occurring sodium, some of these common products are actually processed in some way.

Ask your store manager if nutrition information for unlabeled and locally produced foods is available. If not, following a few general guidelines can make shopping for unlabeled foods a little easier:

PRODUCE If a food is still in its natural "packaging" (for example, whole melons or fresh vegetables), there is less chance that it has been enhanced or changed in the move from farm to market. If a vegetable has been cut, prepared, and commercially packaged, even if it's called "organic" or "natural," there's a possibility that sodium has been added in some form.

POULTRY, MEAT, AND SEAFOOD When choosing among commercial brands, look for unenhanced products, especially uninjected poultry. Although you expect saltwater seafood to contain some naturally occurring sodium, you may be getting more than you bargained for because salt is added to many brands of commercially distributed shrimp, clams, scallops, and mussels. If you're buying local, talk to farmers and distributors to find out how meat has been processed before being brought to market. Keep in mind, too, that locally made sausage, ham, and bacon are just as high in sodium as the commercial brands because salt is needed for the curing process.

BAKED GOODS AND BREADS Bakeries and pastry shops are tempting for a good reason: their products are freshly made and beautifully presented. Just because these treats are not made by a national manufacturer, however, doesn't mean that they are lighter in salt than their commercially distributed counterparts. In fact, most baked goods require a certain amount of salt to rise properly and have a good consistency. You can ask at individual establishments whether nutrition information is available, but these foods are good candidates for the rethink or reduce categories. Save them for occasional treats to save on both sodium and calories.

Decide on Better Alternatives

The best way to make informed purchases is to be a proactive nutrition label reader, then make your choices based on how you plan to use certain foods. Are they something you eat every day, once a week, or only once a month? Can you cut back on the quantity you use if there is no lower-sodium product available? With every purchase, you're deciding how to spend your allotment of dietary sodium. That's why it pays to take your time and think through your selections. Make conscious, educated decisions based on the nutrition facts and on your knowledge of what's most important to you.

Rethink and Eliminate

As you go over your sodium sweep, rethink and decide which high-sodium items you can do without. That's the easiest way of all to cut down on your sodium intake. In Christy's case, the sodium in the packaged side dishes really adds up. She has always relied on a particular brown rice pilaf mix for an easy side dish, but when she sees the cost in sodium that comes with the convenience, she's quick to decide that the cost is too high. She decides instead to cook plain organic brown rice and add her own seasonings that aren't salt based.

Another rethink for Christy is her favorite brand-name frozen Chinese entrée. She has options: she could switch to a lower-sodium brand, but for the biggest impact, she can give up the super-sodium lunch every week and enjoy other favorite ethnic foods at dinner or on weekends instead.

The biggest contributor to Christy's sodium intake is chicken noodle soup. Christy grew up with canned soups as a staple, so she keeps them on hand now as a matter of course. She still loves having soup for lunch, but she decides that canned chicken noodle is one item she and her family can definitely live without. She'd rather try some lower-sodium options or spend a little time making her own healthy soups instead of serving a salty canned soup out of habit. What items in your list can you rethink and do without?

DO WITHOUT . . .	TO SAVE THIS MUCH SODIUM (MG) PER MONTH*
chicken noodle soup at 890 per 1 cup prepared, 2 x per week	7,120
frozen Chinese entrée at 1,350 mg per serving, 1 x per week	5,400
organic brown rice pilaf mix at 530 mg per ½ cup, 2 x per week	4,240
total monthly sodium savings	16,760

*Sodium values have been rounded to the nearest 5 mg.

Replace the High with the Healthy

Manufacturers are tapping into people's interest in reducing sodium and producing many new products with less salt. Look around your grocery store for new options for old favorites and staples. If your usual store doesn't carry low-sodium alternatives, ask your store manager to start stocking them. If you don't get results, try shopping at a store that does.

Sodium content also varies widely from brand to brand. Shrimp is a good example of this variability: the sodium content in frozen packaged shrimp can differ tremendously, depending on the brand. By shopping at a different store than her usual one, Christy finds a brand of frozen shrimp that is processed with three-quarters less salt than the brand she has been buying. Although Christy can replace many of her staple items with commercial low-sodium products, she can also make her own from-scratch versions instead. It's quick and easy to prepare many typically high-sodium sauces, such as cocktail sauce, without adding the high amount of salt found in most processed versions. With these two changes, Christy can transform her sodium-laden shrimp cocktail into a much healthier, much lower sodium, still flavorful dish.

Christy has taken advantage of the obvious savings to be found by simply replacing high-sodium products, in several ways. As illustrated below, she has switched products, going from garlic salt to garlic powder or fresh garlic, and she has switched from regular varieties of products to those with less sodium. You don't have to stick with products labeled "low-salt" or "reduced-salt," either; some brands are just lower in sodium than their counterparts. In addition to these examples, here are some other easy ways to save sodium:

		TO SAVE THIS MUCH SODIUM (MG)*	
REPLACE THIS . . .	**WITH THIS . . .**	**PER SERVING**	**PER MONTH**
garlic salt at 240 per ¼ tsp, 4 x per week	garlic powder or fresh garlic at 0 mg	240	3,840
soy sauce at 1,000 mg per 1 tbsp, 2 x per week	lower-sodium brand at 550 mg	450	3,600
chicken broth at 860 mg per 1 cup, 2 x per week	lower-sodium brand (33% reduced) at 570 mg	290	2,320
shrimp at 805 mg per 3 oz cooked, 2 x per month	shrimp without added brine at 225 mg	580	1,160
black beans at 460 per ½ cup, 1 x per week	lower-sodium brand at 210 mg	250	1,000
cocktail sauce at 760 mg per ¼ cup, 2 x per month	*Cocktail Sauce* (page 172) at 350 mg per ¼ cup	410	820

***Sodium values have been rounded to the nearest 5 mg.**

Reduce How Much or How Often

When you're cooking at home, you have control over how much and how often you eat a certain food or use a certain ingredient. That control gives you the option to continue to use an item you really like and still reduce the amount of sodium it adds to your diet *if* you commit to using less of it or eating it less often. This is a good strategy to pick with, for example, high-sodium dishes that are extra-special favorites or uniquely flavored high-sodium condiments that you simply don't want to do without.

When Christy realizes that she uses high-sodium condiments frequently or in larger than needed amounts, she decides that the easiest way to cut the sodium down to size is to use less rather than give them up.

		TO SAVE THIS MUCH SODIUM (MG)*	
REDUCE THIS . . .	**BY THIS MUCH OR THIS OFTEN . . .**	**PER SERVING**	**PER MONTH**
salsa at 500 mg per ¼ cup, 2 x per week	2 tbsp, 2 x per week	250	2,000
mustard, Dijon, at 360 mg per 1 tbsp, 2 x per week	2 tsp, 2 x per week	120	960
cream of mushroom soup at 830 mg per ½ cup condensed, 2 x per month	1 x per month	830	830
ketchup at 170 mg per 1 tbsp, 3 x per week	1 tbsp, 2 x per week	0 (serving size remains the same)	680

*Sodium values have been rounded to the nearest 5 mg.

Combine Strategies

You are not limited to only one way of cutting back on sodium in the foods you love. In Christy's case, she and her family really like Chinese dishes, but most commercially prepared dishes are just too high in sodium to eat regularly. If the family decides they don't want to do without, however, Christy can do two things: make a delicious home-cooked version for weekly family dinners and buy a lower-sodium frozen brand for an occasional treat. With both strategies, she's effectively lessening the impact of that one dish on her and her family's overall sodium intake.

RETHINK, REPLACE, REDUCE AT HOME

ORIGINAL TOP HIGH-SODIUM FOODS (HIGHEST TO LOWEST)	SODIUM (MG)*	TAKE THIS ACTION . . .	FOR A SAVINGS OF . . .
frozen Chinese entrée (shrimp with garlic sauce)	1,350 per serving	RETHINK: Do without *or* REPLACE: Buy or make a lower-sodium version at 780 mg	**1,350** **570**
frozen Indian entrée (chicken biryani)	1,080 per serving	REDUCE: Buy half as often	**(saving reached over time)**
soy sauce	1,000 per 1 tbsp	REDUCE: Use half as much *or* REPLACE: Buy a lower-sodium brand	**500** **450**
chicken noodle soup, canned, condensed	890 per 1 cup prepared	RETHINK: Do without	**890**
chicken broth, low-fat	860 per 1 cup	REPLACE: Buy a lower-sodium brand *or* make *Chicken Broth* (page 177)	**290** **825**
cream of mushroom soup, canned, condensed	830 per ½ cup condensed	REDUCE: Use less often *or* REPLACE: Buy a lower-sodium brand	**830** **350**
frozen shrimp, large (31–40 count)	805 per 3 oz	REPLACE: Buy a lower-sodium brand	**580**
cocktail sauce	760 per ¼ cup	REPLACE: Make *Cocktail Sauce* (page 172)	**410**
organic brown rice pilaf mix	530 per ½ cup cooked	RETHINK: Do without	**530**
black beans, canned	460 per ½ cup	REPLACE: Buy a lower-sodium brand	**250**

***Sodium values have been rounded to the nearest 5 mg.**

Opposite, you'll find a chart that illustrates how Christy combed her sodium-smart research for 10 of her high-sodium offenders so she could easily consider the best options for her family's lifestyle and food culture.

Watch for High-Sodium Combinations

Cooking at home is a great way to control what you're eating, but unless you're paying attention to the ingredients you use, don't assume that you are automatically creating lower-sodium meals. If your recipe calls for several high-sodium items, you could be serving a homemade dish that's as sodium heavy as a commercial product. Many standard family recipes, such as chili, lasagna, and tuna casserole, contain high-sodium ingredients that together significantly increase the sodium level of the finished dish. Tomatoes and beans are good examples of foods that in themselves do not contain a lot of sodium. When you buy the regular canned products, however, they are processed with salt, significantly increasing the sodium in dishes that call for these foods. Just replacing these staples with lower-sodium options can dramatically cut back on your overall sodium intake.

Take a Stepwise Approach

In the process of assessing your sodium sources, don't let the numbers discourage you. If you're not ready to go to the lowest sodium level right away, choose a product that has less than the one you're using now. Remember that reducing sodium at home is not an all-or-nothing proposition. If using salt-free broth is too extreme for you, switching from regular broth to a 33 percent reduced-sodium version will still move you in the right direction. You can also try combining reduced-sodium and salt-free broths to find a mix that works. If you keep making these small changes, you'll be surprised by how much sodium you can gradually eliminate from your diet.

You don't need to restock your entire kitchen at one time either, although we've provided a list of Sodium-Smart Staples (Part IV, page 260) in case it's helpful. Just stay alert when you shop and keep looking for the best alternative for you at the present time. Many food manufacturers are working toward reducing the sodium in their products, even if they don't make a claim to that effect on their labels. Every so often, recheck nutrition facts labels for your favorite products and be open to new items when they are introduced. As the importance of reducing sodium becomes more widely recognized, you will see more reformulation of food products and the lowering of sodium values. Once you know the facts, it's up to you to decide how to translate them into action.

CHAPTER 6

Identify High-Sodium Foods When Eating Out

Dan's Story: *"My co-workers and I love the food at a nearby Mexican restaurant, and a group of us go there as often as we can after work. A friend of mine kidded me about my diet and asked if I knew what it was doing to my health. It got me thinking just how much sodium and harmful fat really was in all those hefty dishes. The restaurant is a small, family-owned place, so the nutrition information isn't posted anywhere. What could I do? I realized that my favorite dinner—chips and salsa, enchiladas with flour tortillas, rice, and refried beans—was full of ingredients that are high in sodium all on their own. It wasn't hard to figure out that replacing that order with a salad of grilled chicken, lettuce, and avocado with dressing on the side was going to be a better bet for me. I can't totally give up those enchiladas and beans, but I can cut back on how often I order them. When we go out to eat now, I go with the chicken salad half of the time, and I enjoy the food, my friends, and knowing that I'm eating a lot healthier."*

Eating out is a fact of life for most Americans these days, yet whether we find ourselves in restaurants for business, convenience, or pleasure, eating away from home usually also means consuming a lot more sodium than we should.

In a recent review, a consumer watchdog group found that of 102 dishes offered at popular restaurant chains, 85 contained more than a full day's worth of sodium—and some meals contained enough for four days! Even the so-called heart-healthy dishes that on the surface seem like good choices can be shockingly high in sodium.

This "hidden" sodium—along with the excessive amounts of unhealthy fats and sugar that often accompany it—is the reason many restaurant dishes can undermine your best intentions to eat a healthy diet, which is the cornerstone of a healthy lifestyle. In addition to too much sodium, the average American eats too many empty calories from highly processed foods and beverages and not enough calories from the foods that provide good-quality nutrition. Yet if you do a little research and follow the same basics for healthy eating when eating out as when cooking at home—such as knowing which foods offer good nutritional value and choosing wisely—you don't have to compromise your well-being to enjoy the many dining options available. Just use the same three practical strategies of *rethink, replace,* and *reduce* every time you pick up a menu.

SODIUM SHAKEDOWN STRATEGIES

- ✓ Learn how to determine sodium values for restaurant foods.
- ✓ Identify the high-sodium foods and beverages you consume often.
- ✓ Rethink your choices to find the menu items and add-ons you can do without.
- ✓ Replace high-sodium orders with lower-sodium alternatives.
- ✓ Reduce the amount of food you eat and/or the number of times you eat out.

RESEARCH SODIUM SOURCES

Why do most restaurant kitchens serve food with so much sodium, sugar, and unhealthy fats? In large part, it's because restaurant owners and chefs want to please their customers. As Americans' taste buds have become accustomed to saltier-tasting food, chefs have obliged by gradually adding even more salty ingredients, especially salt itself, because customers like it, it makes food taste brighter, and it's very inexpensive.

The ever-growing size of current restaurant portions is also contributing to our high sodium intake. It's a logical outcome: as the amount of food served has increased, so has the amount of sodium eaten.

Because restaurants continue to serve highly salted, high-calorie meals, it would be reasonable to think that eating out less often might be the most effective way to cut back on sodium. However, busy schedules, mobile lifestyles, and the easy availability of restaurant options have made eating out a part of our collective food culture, and that reality is not likely to change much. Fortunately, with a little effort, you can find out how much sodium is in most restaurant dishes, especially at the well-known franchises, and use that information to make educated guesses about the foods served in individually owned establishments as well.

Find the Sodium in Fast-Food and Casual Restaurant Dishes

If you eat out at any of the fast-food places and restaurant chains that are thriving around the country, you should be able to find nutrition information for most of their menu items, either online, at individual locations, or in published resources, such as handy pocket guides. Compare the amount of sodium in your usual choices with other offerings on the menu and see whether you can find lower-sodium options that you'll enjoy.

For most of the dishes in such restaurants, salt and sodium-laden condiments turn simple foods into sodium minefields. For example, a fish fillet on its own isn't high in sodium, but there's plenty of sodium in the salted batter used to bread it for frying. Like the fish fillet, a plain hamburger patty doesn't contain a lot of sodium by itself, but once it's put on a bun and loaded with cheese, ketchup, and pickles—each a highly salted ingredient—that burger becomes a sodium bomb. When you're trying to make healthier choices by comparing nutrition information for menu items, be sure that the numbers you're using include everything on your order—that is, if the numbers are for a hamburger patty, bun, lettuce, tomato, onion, and ketchup, but you add cheese and pickles, you'll also need to include the sodium for these items.

Sauces, salad dressings, and gravies are other major sources of sodium. In most places where the food is made more or less to order, you can ask to have add-ons and extras left off or served on the side. Although fast-food and casual chain restaurants typically take more of an assembly-line approach rather than prepare food from scratch, don't let that stop you from asking for exactly what you want—many restaurants will gladly accommodate your request. The more you can simplify your food by cutting back on extras, the less sodium you'll eat.

Guesstimate the Sodium at Local Restaurants

When you're eating at a restaurant that has created its own menu and doesn't have nutrition information available, you'll need to rely on what you've learned about sources of sodium and your common sense. Every individual establishment prepares its dishes differently, with as much salt and salty products as the chef deems appropriate, so you can't be spot-on when you estimate the sodium in the menu items. In general, though, if you know which ingredients are likely to add up to a high-sodium meal, you can order smarter.

For example, many Italian restaurants serve tomato-based sauces made from high-sodium canned products, and the chefs are likely to use a heavy hand when adding sodium-heavy cheese to many popular dishes. Typical sides, such as salad and garlic bread, may be swathed in salty dressings and toppings. The sodium in these separate items, when combined, can add up very quickly.

Chefs in Asian restaurants frequently use salted stocks and broths and plenty of high-sodium sauces, such as soy sauce. Worsening the sodium problem, soy sauce usually is offered at the table as well. As shown in the story at the start of this chapter, Mexican dishes typically are flavored with salty sauces and cheese, and many include sodium-laden tortillas and chips. To keep your sodium intake lower, order a meal that includes one or two, but not all, of the high-sodium ingredients available. Remember the three R's—*rethink, replace,* and *reduce*—and look for dishes that do not layer sources of sodium.

To discover better alternatives before you order, try to find out as much as you can about how each dish is prepared. Ask questions about spice mixtures, rubs, marinades, and finishing sauces, all of which can be loaded with sodium. If the food is cooked to order, ask the kitchen to use less salt, cheese, or sauce, or whatever other ingredient is likely to be the worst offender, or stick with lightly seasoned main dishes, sides, and salads to which you can add reasonable amounts of sauce or flavorings at the table. As a rule of thumb, simpler dishes contain less sodium than dishes with more ingredients. Soups and combination dishes, such as lasagna or enchiladas, are usually prepared in large batches ahead of time, so it will be too late to ask for less salt or fewer salty ingredients in your order. Also, it is more difficult to reasonably estimate the sodium in the finished product than if you choose simpler, fresher dishes.

Record Your Personal Sodium Sources

As always, tracking and analyzing your own intake is the best way to get an accurate idea of how much sodium is in your food. When you eat out, look up and record the nutrition information for menu items you choose most often, especially at your favorite restaurants. If you created a sodium tracker (see Chapter 3, page 44), you can refer back to capture the meals you recorded. Keep count for at least a month to get a reasonable overview of your typical ordering habits over time.

Take a look at the eating habits of Dan, our single, 27-year-old construction supervisor. He eats out frequently because his job involves a lot of driving around town. He also plays tag football twice a week and likes to go out with his teammates for dinner and a few beers afterward. He doesn't mind cooking at home, but given his schedule and lifestyle, his food choices are more often determined by what's on the menu than by what's in his refrigerator.

MENU ITEM (AS SERVED IN ONE RESTAURANT PORTION)	SODIUM (MG)*
FAST FOOD	
breakfast	
egg-and-sausage biscuit sandwich	1,210
lunch	
¼-lb burger with cheese	1,150
french fries, 3 oz	350
southwestern-style salad with crisp chicken and southwest dressing	1,210
chicken taco salad	1,270
steak burrito	1,110
6-inch cold-cut combo submarine sandwich with 2 tablespoons red wine vinaigrette	1,680
dinner	
Chinese barbecue pork with fried rice	2,130
vegetable and tofu pad Thai	2,680
crispy fried chicken breast with potato salad and biscuit	2,170
pizza, small, cheese with pepperoni and black olives, ½ of pie	1,645
CASUAL DINING	
lunch	
broccoli Cheddar soup, bowl	1,660
California club sandwich with fries	3,950
Greek salad, full portion (1,670 mg), with a cup of French onion soup (1,680 mg)	3,350
boneless Buffalo chicken salad	4,310
grilled ham and Swiss sandwich with fries	4,010
dinner	
"loaded" classic nachos (12)	2,590
beef enchiladas with refried beans and rice	3,790
"lite" chipotle lime chicken	4,990
full order of original ribs	6,510
crispy shrimp tacos	4,760
chicken Parmigiana	3,380

***Sodium values have been rounded to the nearest 5 mg.**
These sample dishes represent actual menu items available at various popular restaurant franchises in the United States, and the nutrition information was taken directly from each establishment's website.

Identify the High-Sodium Menu Items

Once you've identified the menu items you tend to order most when you're eating out, go over the results. Conduct a sodium sweep by circling the dishes and beverages that are highest in sodium, and then make a chart listing them from highest to lowest.

Using the sample menu items from the previous page, here is how Dan's choices stack up:

TOP HIGH-SODIUM MENU ITEMS (HIGHEST TO LOWEST)	SODIUM (MG)*
full order of original ribs	6,510
"lite" chipotle lime chicken	4,990
crispy shrimp tacos	4,760
boneless Buffalo chicken salad	4,310
grilled ham and Swiss sandwich with fries	4,010
California club sandwich with fries	3,950
beef enchiladas with refried beans and rice	3,790
chicken Parmigiana	3,380
Greek salad with a cup of French onion soup	3,350
vegetable and tofu pad Thai	2,680

***Sodium values have been rounded to the nearest 5 mg.**

RETHINK, REPLACE, AND REDUCE

Cutting back on sodium when you're eating out is no different from when you're cooking at home: just put the three sodium-saving strategies—*rethink, replace,* and *reduce*—to work. Start by taking a good, hard look at the highest-sodium items you identified from assessing your own eating habits. What can you do differently to lower the amount of sodium when you eat out? Because of the enormous variety in how restaurant food is prepared, your task is not as simple as comparing labels at the grocery store. However, if you gather reliable nutrition information for your favorite restaurants, you can choose foods with less sodium the next time you stop in. For the places you frequent where nutrition numbers aren't available, you'll have to make an educated guess. The key is to be very attentive to the specifics of the foods you order and diligent in gathering as much information as you can about how dishes are prepared and the ingredients they contain.

Sodium-Smart Planning

Reviewing the food choices you've made in the past provides concrete information you can use to make changes in the future. Using Dan's chart, you can see that he has looked at his top 10 high-sodium meals and decided whether rethinking, replacing, or reducing is the best approach for changing his ways and making healthier choices. You can do the same thing with the record of your own eating habits to make the changes that will have the most impact on your sodium intake.

RETHINK, REPLACE, REDUCE WHEN EATING OUT

ORIGINAL TOP HIGH-SODIUM MENU ITEMS (HIGHEST TO LOWEST)	SODIUM (MG)*	TAKE THIS ACTION . . .	FOR A SAVINGS OF . . .
full order of original ribs	6,510	REDUCE: Choose a half order of ribs (3,800 mg)†	**2,710**
"lite" chipotle lime chicken	4,990	REPLACE: Choose grilled chicken fajitas (1,820 mg)	**3,170**
crispy shrimp tacos	4,760	RETHINK: Eat less often	**(will vary)**
boneless Buffalo chicken salad	4,310	REPLACE: Choose Caribbean-style salad with grilled chicken, dressing on the side (800 mg)	**3,510**
grilled ham and Swiss sandwich with fries	4,010	REDUCE: Choose a lunch-size portion (2,010 mg)†	**2,000**
California club sandwich with fries	3,950	REDUCE: Choose a lunch-size portion (1,970 mg)†	**1,980**
beef enchiladas with refried beans and rice	3,790	REDUCE: Eat less often	**(will vary)**
chicken Parmigiana	3,380	REPLACE: Choose chicken marsala (1,800 mg)	**1,580**
Greek salad with a cup of French onion soup	3,350	RETHINK: Omit the soup (1,680 mg)	**1,670**
vegetable and tofu pad Thai	2,680	RETHINK: Eat less often and never add soy sauce at the table	**(will vary)**

***Sodium values have been rounded to the nearest 5 mg.**
†A smaller or lunch-size order does not contain exactly half the sodium in most cases.

Sodium-Smart Strategies

There will be times when you won't be able to get nutrition information when you eat out. That's when it's useful to remember some general guidelines so that in any situation at any location for almost any dish, you'll have ways to cut back on sodium.

By now you know that some foods generally are higher in sodium than others. Armed with that knowledge, you can order smarter, no matter where you are, by keeping those ingredients to a minimum. Second, it's a no-brainer to know that if you eat less food at a restaurant (or elsewhere), you will almost surely cut down on sodium. When you have little control over what's being served, eating less can be the best option. The third—and simplest—approach of all is to eat out less often. Although that isn't always possible, especially if you're a frequent traveler, it is the one foolproof way to avoid the excessive sodium that, no matter how carefully you choose, is part of most restaurant meals. Regardless of why you eat a high-sodium meal, whether at home or out, you can lessen the impact of the excessive sodium by limiting sodium the rest of that day or the day after.

LIMIT THE HIGH-SODIUM INGREDIENTS THAT ADD UP FAST All the foods below are typically sodium heavy by themselves, so you need to keep them in check. When they are combined, the sodium, of course, piles on. Cut back on dishes that include large amounts of:

- Cheese
- Sauce
- Dressing
- Condiments
- Bread
- Broth and soup
- Processed meat, such as bacon, ham, sausage, and deli meat

AVOID "EXTREME" COMBINATIONS AND SUPER-SIZED PORTIONS The bigger the "wow" factor, the higher the sodium is likely to be. Whenever you're tempted by a menu item that's marketed as bigger and better than usual, steer clear and order the regular but lower-sodium version instead. Even better, order the simplest option with fewer add-ons. Stay away from extreme foods such as:

- Thick-crust, cheese-filled crust, deep-dish, or extra cheesy pizzas
- Super bacon cheeseburgers
- Extra-large orders of fries
- "Loaded" nachos

WATCH FOR WORDING ON MENUS OR NUTRITION ANALYSES THAT COULD BE MISLEADING Remember that just because something is billed as "healthy," it isn't necessarily low in sodium. A large salad with a low-fat dressing can be just as high in sodium as a burger, so don't make assumptions based on catchy phrases or menu claims. Look out for:

- Dishes advertised as healthy, natural, organic, light, low-calorie, gluten-free, or whole-grain; they may or may not be low in sodium
- Portions that include more food than is listed on the nutrition analysis; the information you find on website lists may reflect portions that are different from the plated portion you are actually served, or may not include sides such as french fries or pickles
- Foods analyzed without the usual condiments, sauces, or dressings; be sure to include everything you eat when you tally the sodium content

MAKE THE BETTER CHOICES AS OFTEN AS YOU CAN Wherever you are and whatever the options, you can always go for the one that offers the most nutrition with the least added salt. For sodium-savvy suggestions, try these:

- Choose steamed rice over fried rice, pilaf, or other flavored rice dishes.
- Go to the salad bar and create your own, including a combination of low-sodium toppings, instead of ordering a stock salad from the menu that includes high-sodium items. If there is no salad bar, see if the kitchen will prepare a simple salad with dressing on the side for you.
- Frequent restaurants where food is prepared to order and ask for lower-sodium dishes, such as steamed vegetables without margarine or salt added in the kitchen. You can always add a sprinkling of salt at the table, if needed.
- Be innovative. If the menu lists something that sounds good to you but is likely to be high in sodium, you can ask for it to be served in a lower-sodium way. For example, instead of ordering the green salad with marinated or crispy chicken as listed, you might be able to substitute plain grilled chicken as the salad topper.

Eating away from home without eating too much sodium can certainly pose a challenge, but you don't need to put your good food sense on the back burner. If restaurant and take-out meals are part of your established food culture, learn how to manage the menus to your advantage. When you are trying to balance eating out with eating healthy, find the combination of *rethink, replace,* and *reduce* that works best for you. By doing so, you can continue to enjoy eating out without compromising your commitment to lower your sodium.

CHAPTER 7

Stay Focused on Eating Well

Dorothy's Story: *"I've been trying to lose weight for as long as I can remember, and I've always focused on how to cut calories. But I honestly never thought much about whether I was getting good nutrition from the low-calorie foods I ate. I found out last year that I had high blood pressure, and I became concerned about both the calories and the salt in my diet. Now I watch for high-sodium foods* and *try to pay attention to how my choices add up nutritionally. I know I'm eating better, and I feel a lot better for it!"*

The cornerstone of a healthy lifestyle is maintaining nutritious eating habits, and consuming a limited amount of sodium is an important piece of an overall heart-healthy diet. Yet to feed your body properly, you need a full spectrum of nutrients, minerals, and fiber. For the greatest health benefit, include the recommended combinations of all the food groups and eat portions that allow you to maintain a healthy weight.

EAT WELL STRATEGIES

✓ Establish eating habits that nourish your body and keep you healthy.
✓ Focus on foods that are high in the nutrients your body needs.
✓ Limit foods that are low in nutrients but high in sodium, saturated and trans fats, cholesterol, added sugar, and empty calories.
✓ Eat reasonable portions to reduce both calorie and sodium consumption.
✓ Follow heart-healthy diet recommendations both at home and when you eat out.

HIGH NUTRITION, LOWER SODIUM

The link between good nutrition and good health is clear: eating well over time will improve your odds of living longer without developing chronic risk factors and health problems. On the other hand, living on foods that are low in nutrients increases your risk of heart disease and other conditions that can lessen the quality of your life. The following strategies will help you work toward improving your overall diet as you also begin to lower your sodium intake.

Make Good Food Choices

Making good food choices every day will add up over time to keep your body well nourished and at a healthy weight.

- Eat a wide variety of nutritious foods in the right amounts from all the food groups.
  - » Include lots of different kinds of vegetables and fruits, especially the deeply colored ones.
  - » Choose fat-free, 1 percent, and low-fat dairy products.
  - » Include plenty of fiber-rich, whole-grain foods.
  - » Eat fish, preferably fish containing omega-3 fatty acids (for example, salmon, trout, and tuna), at least twice a week.
  - » Select lean meats and skinless poultry.
  - » Include legumes, nuts, and seeds.
  - » Choose healthy fats and oils.
- Limit foods that are high in calories but low in nutrients.
  - » Limit beverages and foods with added sugars that provide zero nutrients.
  - » Reduce the amount of saturated fat, trans fat, and cholesterol you eat.
  - » Keep sodium to a minimum by choosing unprocessed foods and products that are the lowest sodium available, and by using little or no salt when preparing foods.
  - » If you drink alcohol, drink in moderation.

Eat a Wide Variety of Nutritious Foods

To achieve a good balance of nutrients in your meals, try to eat a variety of choices from each of the seven categories of food discussed in this section. If you eat only the same few foods over and over, you may not get enough of some of the nutrients you need—and you'll get bored. Instead of getting stuck in a rut, try new things and experiment with interesting combinations. Good food is one of life's pleasures, and eating for good health, with less sodium, can be delicious and satisfying.

VEGETABLES AND FRUITS Try lots of different veggies and fruits, and use them in main dishes as well as for nutritious sides. Fresh, frozen, or canned, they provide a broad range of nutrients, including vitamins, minerals, and fiber. Focus especially on the deeply colored choices since these tend to contain the most nutrients. Good vegetable picks include tomatoes, beets, sweet potatoes, broccoli, and bell peppers; nutrient-rich fruits include strawberries, blueberries, oranges, and pineapple.

> **BE SODIUM SMART:** Watch for the sodium in "regular" canned vegetables. Although these foods are packed with good nutrition, they are almost always full of salt as well. Look for no-salt-added or low-sodium options instead; rinsing canned produce can help remove some of the sodium.

FAT-FREE, 1 PERCENT, AND LOW-FAT DAIRY PRODUCTS Milk and milk-based foods provide important nutrients, especially calcium and protein, but full-fat dairy products are also high in saturated fat and cholesterol. To get all the goodness and health benefits of dairy foods, such as milk, yogurt, sour cream, and cheeses, including cottage cheese, choose fat-free, 1 percent, and low-fat products whenever possible.

> **BE SODIUM SMART:** Some dairy foods are surprisingly high in sodium. Salt is needed to make most cheeses, including cottage cheese, so these products typically contain more sodium than you might think. Be sure to compare nutrition facts panels and look for products that are low in fat *and* sodium.

FIBER-RICH WHOLE GRAINS Because they are filling and offer many nutritious benefits, grains have long been a mainstay of many food cultures around the world. In addition to providing a variety of nutrients, whole grains offer both soluble and insoluble fiber. (Grains that are not processed to remove the grain kernel are considered whole.) Eating enough fiber from whole grains can help reduce blood cholesterol levels, and because grains leave you feeling more satisfied, they can assist you in controlling your weight as well. Try to eat whole-grain versions of at least half of your breads, pastas, rice, and other grains. In addition to well-known grains such as wheat and corn, try bulgur, farro, barley, and quinoa for some variety and whole-grain goodness, but stay away from seasoned mixes that add a lot of sodium.

> **BE SODIUM SMART:** The amounts of sodium in breads, crackers, and cereals vary widely, depending on the type and the manufacturer. Compare nutrition facts panels and try different products until you find the varieties that satisfy both your taste buds and your sodium needs.

FISH RICH IN OMEGA-3 FATTY ACIDS Seafood is an excellent source of protein, and eating fish varieties that contain high levels of heart-healthy omega-3 fatty acids can help you reduce your risk of heart disease. Examples of such fish are salmon, tuna, and trout.

BE SODIUM SMART: Using canned tuna is an inexpensive and easy way to increase your omega-3 intake, but try to steer clear of products that are high in sodium. To enjoy the tuna without the salt, look for the very low sodium options that are now available.

LEAN MEATS AND SKINLESS POULTRY Despite the penchant many Americans have for meat and poultry, most adults don't need more than 3 to 6 ounces cooked weight (4 to 8 ounces when raw) each day for good health. To avoid consuming a lot of saturated fat and cholesterol, stick with lean cuts of meat (sirloin, tenderloin, and eye of round, for example) and skinless poultry (chicken and turkey breast meat and tenderloin, for example).

BE SODIUM SMART: Processed meats, such as ham, sausage, frankfurters, and deli meats, all contain large amounts of added sodium. Limit these foods to two servings a week instead of using them as part of your regular routine, and check nutrition facts panels to find the lowest-sodium products. Also, watch out for fresh chicken, turkey, and pork that have been enhanced with a salt-containing solution or brine; when you see statements such as "self-basting" or "contains up to __% of __," it means that a sodium-containing solution has been added to the product. Even the phrase "natural flavor" can be a tip that brine has been added.

LEGUMES, NUTS, AND SEEDS Legumes, the class of food that includes beans and peas (both are the mature forms of legume), as well as lentils, are excellent sources of plant protein. They also provide other nutrients, such as iron and zinc, in amounts similar to those in meats, poultry, and fish, and they are rich in dietary fiber and potassium, which help keep blood pressure low. In addition to lentils, common legumes include dried beans (kidney, pinto, black, lima, and others), dried peas (split, black-eyed, and chickpeas), and peanuts. Nuts and seeds are rich in unsaturated fats, which can help reduce blood pressure and harmful cholesterol; remember, though, that nuts are also high in calories.

BE SODIUM SMART: Because legumes taste rather bland unless well seasoned, most mixed dishes that include them use some kind of sauce for flavor. As you should do anytime you use a sauce, watch for added sodium that can turn a sodium-smart food into a salt trap. Be sure, too, to use unsalted nuts and seeds.

HEALTHY FATS AND OILS The unsaturated fats found in vegetable oils provide essential nutrients and are part of a balanced diet. Whenever possible, use those oils and other unsaturated fats, such as light tub margarine, instead of either animal-based fats high in saturated fat, such as butter, or margarines that contain trans fat. All fats are high in calories, so use even the healthy ones in moderation.

> **BE SODIUM SMART:** Healthy oils, such as canola, olive, corn, and safflower, and cooking sprays don't contain sodium, but manufactured fats, such as margarine, do. Although fat-free spray margarine doesn't provide the nutrients of oils, it is an unsaturated, low-calorie alternative to saturated and trans fats. Compare nutrition facts labels to find the product that is lowest in saturated fat, trans fat, and sodium.

> **QUICK REFERENCE TO GOOD NUTRITION GOALS**
>
> *For a 2,000-calorie daily diet, aim for:*
>
> - **VEGETABLES:** 4 to 5 servings a day
> - **FRUITS:** 4 to 5 servings a day
> - **FAT-FREE, 1 PERCENT, AND LOW-FAT DAIRY PRODUCTS:** 2 to 3 servings a day
> - **FIBER-RICH WHOLE GRAINS:** 6 to 8 servings a day
> - **FISH RICH IN OMEGA-3 FATTY ACIDS:** 2 servings a week
> - **LEAN MEATS AND SKINLESS POULTRY:** a *limit of* 3 to 6 (cooked) ounces a day depending on calorie needs
> - **LEGUMES, NUTS, AND SEEDS:** 4 to 5 servings a week
> - **HEALTHY FATS AND OILS:** 2 to 3 servings a day if calorie needs allow
>
> For a handy reference chart of what constitutes a healthy serving for each food group, see "Food Groups and Suggested Servings" in the Toolkit (Part IV, page 262).

Focus on Key Nutrients

Several essential nutrients found in whole foods work together to regulate blood pressure, and it is important to get enough of these in your diet.

POTASSIUM Potassium blunts the effect of sodium on blood pressure and plays a critical part in helping the body excrete excess sodium to keep the level of sodium regulated and balanced. Potassium also is needed for proper muscle function. It helps the muscle tissue in the walls of arteries and other blood vessels relax, which in turn allows blood vessels to open, or dilate. This allows blood to flow more easily and keeps blood pressure lower, much in the same way that certain medications (vasodilators) work.

- The recommended goal for adults is to consume about 4,700 mg of potassium each day, yet most of us eating a typical American diet get less than half of that amount.
- Good sources of potassium include potatoes (both white and sweet), white beans, bananas, dried apricots, yogurt (fat-free, plain), spinach, and certain fish (such as Atlantic salmon, halibut, yellowfin tuna, and trout).

CALCIUM Calcium helps regulate blood pressure through its role both in the contraction and relaxation of the smooth muscle cells in artery walls and in reducing blood volume.

- The recommended daily intake for calcium is 1,000 mg a day for adults ages 19 to 50; after 50, it's 1,200 mg. Many people, however, do not get enough calcium.
- Good sources of calcium include fortified cereals, fat-free or low-fat milk and cheese, greens (such as turnip, collard, and beet), and soybeans. Following a heart-healthy diet and eating the recommended servings of fat-free dairy products will provide at least 1,000 mg of calcium daily.

MAGNESIUM Magnesium is another important component for blood pressure regulation. It is needed for the production of an essential lipid compound that causes blood vessels to relax and widen. Magnesium also works to keep the levels of sodium, potassium, and calcium properly balanced within cells.

- The recommended daily intake of magnesium is 400 mg, but as happens with potassium and calcium, few people get this amount from their diet.
- Good sources of magnesium include spinach, seeds (such as pumpkin, sunflower, and sesame), whole grains (such as quinoa, buckwheat flour, bulgur, and oat bran), and small amounts of unsalted nuts (such as almonds, pine nuts, and walnuts).

FIBER Fiber is broken down into two types: soluble in water and insoluble in water. Both are indigestible complex carbohydrates, but they have different effects in the body. Soluble fiber is involved in the regulation of several body processes, including the production of cholesterol and glucose. Insoluble fiber contributes bulk that provides a feeling of fullness and helps food and waste move through the digestive system. Most foods contain both types of fiber in varying proportions.

- Good sources of fiber include beans (such as navy, kidney, black, pinto, lima, and cannellini), bran cereals, lentils, split peas, and pears.

- The recommended daily intake of fiber for men is 30 to 35 grams; women should aim for 20 to 25 grams. Children need fiber, too, and should get about 14 grams in every 1,000 calories they eat in a day.

CUT BACK ON EMPTY CALORIES AND UNHEALTHY FATS

Sodium isn't the only thing that can put your health at risk if you eat too much of it. You also can eat too many empty calories—that is, calories that do not add nutrients to food. You'll find empty calories in added sugar and solid fat (in the form of saturated and trans fats). (See page 96 for examples of added sugar's "aliases.") Empty calories contribute to weight gain, which can increase your risk of high blood pressure, diabetes, and heart disease. As you work to lower the amount of sodium you consume, keep in mind that you need to limit these other two dietary health hazards, too.

Examples of popular foods and beverages that provide most of the empty calories for Americans include:

- Cakes, cookies, pastries, doughnuts, and candy (which contain both solid fat and added sugar)
- Sodas, energy drinks, sports drinks, and fruit drinks (which contain added sugar)
- Full-fat cheeses (which contain solid fat)
- Pizza (which contains solid fat)
- Ice cream (which contains both solid fat and added sugar)
- Sausages, hot dogs, bacon, and ribs (which contain solid fat)

Most of us already know that the examples such as candy and soda have no nutritional value and are sources of empty calories. In some cases, however, even foods that provide important nutrients also contain empty calories that are added in food preparation (at home or away) or manufacturing. Examples include sweetened cereals (added sugar) and fried chicken (saturated fat from frying and from eating the skin). Although it is important to limit empty calories, eating a small amount may fit within your particular calorie and nutrient needs and still let you follow an overall healthy eating plan. Most people eat *far more* empty calories than they need or is healthy, however.

You can lower your intake of empty calories by following the same strategies you're using to limit sodium: *rethink, replace,* and *reduce.* For example, you could decide that you don't really need to have a bowl of ice cream every evening; if you can't go cold turkey and give it up, eat half a bowl or buy ice cream packaged in single servings to make portion control easy. Perhaps you'll choose to replace foods that contain added sugar or solid fat with healthier versions, such as by switching from fruit drinks to 100 percent fruit juices or from regular sodas to diet sodas to eliminate the added sugar. You could also choose to replace full-fat cheeses with the fat-free and low-fat varieties. Be sure to check that your replacement foods actually contain fewer calories, and no more sodium, than the regular versions you were consuming.

Keep Added Sugar to a Minimum

The sugar in your diet can be naturally occurring or added. Naturally occurring sugars are found in foods such as fruit (fructose) and milk (lactose). Added sugars are sugars and syrups put in foods during preparation or processing or at the table, contributing only empty calories. In addition to the soft drinks, desserts, and snacks listed on page 95, other sweetened dairy products, such as flavored yogurt and chocolate milk, and sweetened grains, such as cinnamon toast and honey-nut waffles, are common sources of added sugar.

For packaged foods, the nutrition facts panel combines natural and added sugars into a total amount, given in total grams. Each gram contains 4 calories, so if a product has 15 grams of sugar per serving, that's 60 calories just from the sugar.

To tell whether a processed food contains added sugar, look at the list of ingredients. Besides sugar itself, words that indicate added sugar include those ending in *ose,* such as *maltose* or *sucrose,* and high *fructose* corn syrup, molasses, cane sugar, corn sweetener, raw sugar, syrup, honey, and fruit juice concentrates.

In general, most American women should aim to limit the amount of added sugar to no more than 100 calories per day, or about 6 teaspoons of added sugar. Men should aim for no more than 150 calories per day, or about 9 teaspoons. Compare those numbers with the sugar in just one 12-ounce can of regular soda: 8 teaspoons of sugar, or 130 calories, with no nutritional value at all. As a guideline, both men and women should try to limit sugar-sweetened beverages to no more than 450 calories a week.

To reduce the amount of added sugar—and empty calories—in your diet, try these sugar-zapping tips:

- Cut back on the amount of sugar you add to things you eat or drink regularly, such as cereal and coffee or tea. Wean yourself from using too much by cutting your usual amount of sugar by half, then using even less or none if you can, or switch to an artificial sweetener.

- Try nonnutritive sweeteners, such as aspartame, sucralose, or saccharin, in moderation. (The Food and Drug Administration has determined that these sweeteners are safe, and they may help you satisfy your sweet tooth without adding calories to your diet.)
- Buy sugar-free or low-calorie beverages.
- Buy fresh fruits, unsweetened frozen fruits, or fruits canned in water or natural juice. Avoid sweetened frozen fruits and fruits canned in syrup, especially heavy syrup.
- Sweeten your cereals by adding fruit or sweet spices, such as cinnamon, instead of sugar.
- Cut back on the sugar in recipes and add extracts, such as almond, vanilla, orange, or lemon, for a flavor boost.

Limit the Harmful Fats in Your Diet

An easy way to tell whether a fat is the kind that provides empty calories and is harmful to your health is to see whether it stays solid at room temperature. If so, it contains saturated fat and/or trans fat. Eating a diet that is high in saturated fat and trans fat can increase your chance of developing high blood cholesterol, which in turn increases your risk of heart disease. Saturated fat is found in animal-based foods, such as dairy products (butter, whole milk, and full-fat cheese, for example) and meat and poultry. Some tropical oils (coconut, palm, and palm kernel) also contain high amounts of saturated fat. To protect your heart, keep your intake of saturated fat to less than 7 percent of your total daily calories; for a 2,000-calorie intake, that would be 140 calories, or about 16 grams of saturated fat.

Trans fat has been used in many commercial products, especially baked goods, fried foods, and stick margarine; this fat results from hydrogenation, the process that makes liquid oils more solid. Because trans fat may be the most damaging of the harmful fats, it is recommended that you eat as little as possible (no more than 1 percent of total daily calories).

Like saturated and trans fats, dietary cholesterol, another type of fat from animal sources, can increase blood cholesterol; therefore, it's wise to limit how much dietary cholesterol you eat. The current recommendation is no more than 300 mg a day. You can find the amount of cholesterol, as well as saturated and trans fats, in processed foods by reading the nutrition facts panels. To cut back on the fats that can hurt your heart, replace them as often as possible with healthy, unsaturated oils. Good examples include canola, corn, olive, safflower, and sunflower oils.

MAKE EATING WELL A LIFESTYLE PRIORITY

If you decide that your current eating habits need a makeover, rest assured that you're not alone. Many of us who juggle the demands of busy lifestyles end up choosing convenience and speed over better health. Don't fret over past food choices—just commit now to changing what you can so you can stick to a nutritious and delicious eating plan and adopt new behaviors for the rest of your life.

Size Up Your Servings

Portion control is an essential strategy for both sodium reduction and weight management. If you keep your servings in line, you'll be able to more easily keep your intake of sodium under control—even when eating out or enjoying high-sodium favorites at home. For a guide, refer to "Food Groups and Suggested Servings" in the Toolkit (Part IV, page 262).

Given the huge portions that most restaurants serve these days, it is hard to know what a reasonable serving should look like. Use these comparisons as a guide: a deck of cards is about the size of a serving of meat or poultry, and a checkbook is about the size of a serving of fish. A baseball makes a good guide for a 1-cup serving of dairy, for example, and it's also about the same size as a medium piece of fruit. Imagine a billiard ball when portioning out a ½-cup serving, and a Ping-Pong ball for about 2 tablespoons.

Understand Your Triggers

Why do we eat so much if we know that overeating isn't good for us? Scientists are actively studying the psychology of portion distortion, and their research has yielded some interesting observations about our seemingly irrational behavior. To start with, the fact is that good nutrition is a long-term goal, but for most people, daily food choices provide enjoyment in the short term. Therefore, to receive a payback that is years away, we need to be able to delay satisfaction now; for most of us, that is hard to do.

Research has identified other factors that also play into the dynamic and shift the focus of our decision making to "now" versus "later." When foods are easily available, attractive visually and/or economically, and offer immediate gratification, we are much more likely to make choices, and eat amounts of food, that we *know* are not consistent with what we believe is healthy. The internal thinking goes, *I'm hungry; I'm busy; that food is right here. I'll eat it now and deal with the consequences later.*

The results of these studies have led to some good suggestions for keeping the amount of food we eat in check. Effective strategies include:

- Making food choices in advance and mentally locking them in as defaults
- Practicing "conscious" eating, which means staying aware of *why* you are eating
- Eating on a smaller plate so the amount of food looks greater and more satisfying
- Waiting at least 20 minutes after eating to allow your brain to register that your stomach is full before you eat more

Eat Smart When Eating Out

Dining out can put your best intentions to the test, especially if you're trying to cut back on sodium; but if you keep the basic guidelines for good nutrition in mind, you can enjoy a restaurant meal without compromising your good health. Review the strategies in Chapter 6, "Identify High-Sodium Foods When Eating Out," on how to make good choices in restaurants.

Try these other general eating-out tips:

- Ask questions so you know exactly how a dish is prepared.
- Request that your food be prepared without add-ons and salt.
- Choose foods that are grilled, broiled, steamed, or baked instead of fried.
- Find out whether your selection can be prepared in a healthier way if it typically is fried; if the food has a sauce, ask for it on the side.
- Order dishes that offer vegetables and whole grains instead of lots of meat or poultry to increase fiber and cut down on calories and fat.
- Split an entrée with your dining partner or put half in a take-home container before you start to eat your meal.

The three "R" strategies—*rethink, replace,* and *reduce*—apply as much to making other more nutritious food choices as to reducing sodium. To revamp your eating habits, identify what you'd like to eliminate or change and how you can reduce the quantity while improving the quality of the food you eat. To help you make those transitions, Chapter 8, "Plan Ahead with Lower-Sodium Menus," provides simple guidelines and a sample lower-sodium menu plan so you can create your own healthy menus that fit your lifestyle and satisfy your food preferences. In Part III, you'll also find more than 60 recipes that are low in sodium as well as delicious and heart healthy.

CHAPTER 8

Plan Ahead with Lower-Sodium Menus

Christy's Story: *"I've always wanted to provide my family with the best of everything, and that includes healthy, low-sodium meals. As soon as I became aware of the health consequences of a high-sodium diet, I was on a mission and really worked to lower our sodium intake. But after a while, I gradually slipped back into my old habits. I guess I just 'forgot' to keep track of sodium as much. I knew I needed a way to control our sodium intake without having to think about it all the time. A neighbor suggested that I do what she does—write out a fixed plan for one week and refuse to buy anything that isn't on it. Using the kitchen inventory I'd made when sodium was a top priority, I had no trouble making a detailed list of the foods I needed for a week's worth of meals. With no decisions left to make, it was easier for me to stick to my commitment to cut back on sodium. Having a written plan certainly did the trick for me!"*

Planning ahead can be a huge help in making lower-sodium choices a permanent part of your everyday routine. Having an entire week's worth of planned meals that don't go over your sodium budget frees you from having to make quick calculations and on-the-spot decisions. Knowing in advance what to buy at the store or order at a restaurant also protects you from temptations that can derail your best intentions.

Perhaps most important, following an established eating plan allows you to take the time you need to let your palate adjust to tasting less salt. Plan to decrease your current sodium intake in gradual increments, one step at a time. It can take from six weeks to six months for your taste buds to completely adapt, but the more often you repeat your healthy choices, the more you will reinforce your commitment to reduce the sodium in your diet. As the saying goes, repeat an action 30 times and it becomes habit. In your case, make the same lower-sodium choice 30 times and you'll establish a pattern that stays with you for life.

Following a defined eating plan also gives you better control over the nutritional quality of what you eat. Whether you're using a professionally developed eating plan or creating your own, you're more likely to focus on the long-term benefits of eating well than give in to an impulsive and unhealthy splurge. To make your lower-sodium planning more interesting, experiment with new flavors and healthy cooking techniques to personalize your meals.

LOWER-SODIUM MENU PLANNING STRATEGIES

✓ Understand how to maximize nutrition and budget your sodium intake with a balanced eating plan.

✓ Create your own healthy, lower-sodium eating plan or follow our suggested plan.

✓ Experiment with sodium-free seasonings and natural flavorings to perk up what you eat.

✓ Use heart-healthy cooking techniques and tips to create delicious lower-sodium meals at home.

CREATING A LOWER-SODIUM EATING PLAN

Creating your own meal plans gives you control over what you eat and focuses your attention on your long-term goals. With a plan in hand, you'll eat healthier food, experience less backsliding, and be less likely to give in to temptation. Smart planning also allows you to shop and cook more efficiently, so you can save both time and money. Because you're making the decisions up front, you can focus on good food that delivers quality nutrition and is prepared just the way you like it.

The three major elements of a heart-smart eating plan are:

- The right balance of foods to provide *adequate nutrition*
- The *right calorie count* to meet your body's needs
- A *lower-sodium intake* that doesn't exceed a healthy level

Make Your Calories Count

The first goal when drawing up a meal plan is to combine the foods that provide balanced nutrition at a calorie level that is right for you. Using the information in Chapter 7, which covers the basics of eating right for good health, decide how to include each food group and tailor the servings to meet your needs.

Standardized dietary guidelines estimate that healthy adults need an average of 2,000 calories a day; an ideal eating plan would include:

EACH DAY:

- ✓ 4 to 5 servings (or 2½ cups total) of vegetables (VG)
- ✓ 4 to 5 servings (or 2½ cups total) of fruit (FR)
- ✓ 6 to 8 servings of grain products (GR), preferably whole grain
- ✓ 2 to 3 servings of dairy products (DA)
- ✓ 2 servings of protein (PRO), such as meat, poultry, seafood, or vegetarian sources
- ✓ Up to 2 servings of healthy fats and oils (FAT) if calorie needs allow

EACH WEEK:

- ✓ 2 to 3 servings of nuts and seeds (NUT) if calorie needs allow
- ✓ 2 to 3 servings of legumes (LEG)

The sample menu plans in this chapter are based on that daily average of 2,000 calories, but everyone has individual needs. If you are a petite woman who requires fewer total calories to maintain a healthy weight, your calorie breakdown should reflect that in every food category. On the other hand, if you're an active 6 foot 6 inch man, your calorie needs will be higher. To find out how many servings are recommended for different calorie intakes, see "Food Groups and Suggested Servings" in the Toolkit (Part IV, page 262).

There are many ways to combine daily servings from each food group to reach about 2,000 calories. Here's one suggestion:

SAMPLE FOOD GROUP COMBINATIONS		CALORIES—AIM FOR
breakfast	1 grain, 1 dairy, 1 fruit, 1 fat	about 450
snack	1 dairy, 1 fruit	about 200
lunch	1 protein, 2 grain, 2 vegetable	about 500
snack	1 dairy, 1 grain, 1 fruit	about 250
dinner	1 protein, 2 grain, 2 vegetable, 1 fruit, 1 fat	about 600
	total	**about 2,000**

Budget Your Sodium Intake

As you do with calories, you need to know how much sodium you can allot in your personal eating plan. Unlike with calories, however, you don't get more sodium because you are taller and/or more active and therefore need more nutrients!

Think of sodium in terms of a budget: you have so much to spend each day, and you have total freedom to spend it any way you like; once that amount is used up, you're overdrawn on your account. Just as you decide how much money you can spend on rent, food, and other necessities each month, you can establish a budget to manage your sodium intake each day.

But how do you know how much sodium you can "spend" in the first place? According to the American Heart Association's recommendations for best health, you should budget for a daily maximum of 1,500 mg. The breakdown might look like this:

	SODIUM (MG)—AIM FOR
breakfast	350
snack	100
lunch	450
snack	100
dinner	500
total	**1,500**

If you're not ready to try for that daily goal yet, you can set one or even two interim target goals. The easiest way to start is to refer to the information you recorded in your initial sodium tracker. To decide on your first goal, you could take your daily average intake from your tracker and reduce it by one-fourth. For example, the average intake taken from the series of sample trackers in Chapter 3 is just under 5,200 mg per day, and three-fourths of that equals about 3,900 mg. However, these examples are intended to represent very high sodium profiles and are higher than national averages. Your own tracker will likely show a more typical sodium intake of about 3,400 mg a day. Multiply your average by 0.75 for your initial daily target; using the example of about 3,400 mg, the result would be about 2,550 mg for the target. As you make progress in lowering your sodium and achieving your best health, you'll want to continue lowering your goal.

Assuming that you're just starting to transition to a lower-sodium diet, try aiming for a compromise daily target of about 2,300 mg. Based on your habits, decide how much sodium is reasonable for each meal. For example, if you know you eat a light breakfast every day but usually eat out for lunch, you'll want to allot less sodium for breakfast and more for the midday meal. (Don't forget to use some of the total for snacks and medications, depending on your needs.) For example, you could plan on allowing 500 mg of sodium for breakfast, 750 mg for lunch, and 750 mg for dinner, leaving up to 300 mg to "spend" on extras. If you eat snacks, you could assign two snacks a day at 250 mg each, leaving 1,800 mg to divide among your three meals. Having a preset number in mind as you make decisions each day will help you estimate what you have left to spend in your sodium budget. When you do eat a high-sodium meal, such as at a favorite restaurant where you always meet friends for dinner on Fridays, plan to allow extra sodium for the restaurant food and eat less sodium at breakfast and lunch that day.

In the example below, you can see that lunch on this day far exceeds the amount of sodium allotted for a daily target goal of 2,300 mg. Even so, if you scale back on other meals to compensate, it's certainly possible to stay in range of your target goal.

	TARGET SODIUM GOAL (MG)	ACTUAL SODIUM INTAKE (MG)
breakfast	450	400
snack	200	125
lunch	550	1,250
snack	200	25
dinner	700	400
medications (if applicable)	200	200
total	**2,300**	**2,400**

Find the Right Combination of Nutrition, Calories, and Sodium

Using the suggested breakdowns of healthy foods, calories, and sodium, you're ready to create your own meal plans. If you were to base your target plan on an ideal intake of 2,000 calories and the interim step of 2,300 mg of sodium, here is a possible scenario:

SAMPLE FOOD GROUP COMBINATIONS		CALORIES—AIM FOR	SODIUM (MG)—AIM FOR
breakfast	1 grain, 1 dairy, 1 fruit, 1 fat	about 450	about 450
snack	1 dairy, 1 fruit	about 200	about 200
lunch	1 protein, 2 grain, 2 vegetable	about 500	about 550
snack	1 dairy, 1 grain, 1 fruit	about 250	about 200
dinner	1 protein, 2 grain, 2 vegetable, 1 fruit, 1 fat	about 600	about 700
	Medications (if applicable)	0	about 200
	total	**2,000**	**2,300**

Create a similar chart using your own parameters, and refer to it as a guide when you're deciding what foods to buy and how to combine them when you're planning meals. You can use the blank Daily Menu Planner template (Part IV, page 255) provided in the Toolkit to get started. By doing a little up-front planning, you'll have the flexibility to create a personalized plan that reflects both the ways you eat and the demands of your own lifestyle *and* concretely lowers your sodium intake. The variables are infinite; it's up to you to find the combinations that work best for the way you live.

FOLLOWING A DEFINED EATING PLAN

Even though sodium is so abundant in today's food supply, you *can* find ways to cut back. If, however, staying aware of the need to make lower-sodium food choices every day feels like a grind, you may prefer using an established menu plan that takes out the guesswork and does the thinking for you. As a result, you may find it easier to stick to the sodium-savvy plan longer and therefore cement good eating habits into routine.

If you'd like some ideas on how to get started, look over the three-day meal plans that follow. These plans are loosely based on the sample tracker and pantry sweep of Christy, the mom you read about in Chapters 3 and 5 (pages 31 and 60). See how these menus fit with your typical eating habits and lifestyle; make tweaks as needed, then give the menus a try. Following a defined plan that automatically provides the nutrients you need and keeps the sodium low will give your taste buds a chance to adapt and your brain an opportunity to relax as you transition to a healthier diet.

All the foods included in this first step-down plan are store-bought unless otherwise specified; we've even included one restaurant meal. To start the transition to a lower-sodium diet, Christy has replaced her high-sodium deli meats and rice mixes with the recipes for Roasted Turkey (page 160) and Veggie Mac and Cheese (page 192) in this book. For busy days and nights, though, we've also provided lower-sodium choices that don't involve preparing a special recipe.

CHRISTY'S FIRST STEP-DOWN MENU PLAN AT 2,000 CALORIES AND 2,300 MG SODIUM

DAY 1 AT 2,300 MG SODIUM	CALORIES	SODIUM (MG)*	FOOD GROUP
breakfast			
1¼ cups shredded wheat minis with	170	0	2½ GR
8 oz fat-free milk	85	105	1 DA
½ cup blueberries	40	0	1 FR
1 tbsp chopped walnuts, unsalted	50	0	
subtotal	**345**	**105**	
snack			
2 tbsp low-sodium peanut butter	200	65	1 NUT
1 medium banana	105	0	1 FR
subtotal	**305**	**65**	
lunch			
sandwich of			
2 slices low-sodium whole-grain bread	140	200	2 GR
3 oz *Roasted Turkey* (page 160) or equal amount of plain chicken breast	135	45	1 PRO
½ cup chopped romaine and 3 slices tomato	10	5	1 VG
2 tsp honey mustard	20	50	
8 oz iced tea, unsweetened	0	0	
subtotal	**305**	**300**	

DAY 1 AT 2,300 MG SODIUM	CALORIES	SODIUM (MG)*	FOOD GROUP
snack			
1½ oz low-fat Colby cheese	75	265	1 DA
6 low-fat, whole-grain crackers	120	160	1 GR
½ cup green grapes	60	0	1 FR
subtotal	**255**	**425**	
dinner			
2 frozen crunchy breaded fish fillets with	240	550	1 PRO
2 tbsp tartar sauce	80	250	1 FAT
1 cup green beans, no-salt-added canned	40	20	2 VG
½ cup *Veggie Mac and Cheese* (page 192) or equal amount of plain pasta with light tub margarine and herbs	100	160	1 GR
2 cups mixed salad greens	20	30	2 VG
2 tbsp low-fat oil and vinegar dressing	70	200	1 FAT
4 oz white wine	100	5	
1 *Luscious Lemon Sponge Pudding* (page 248)	195	90	½ FR
subtotal	**845**	**1,305**	
totals	2,055	2,200	**5 VG, 3½ FR, 6½ GR, 2 DA, 2 PRO, 2 FAT, 1 NUT**

Note: GR indicates grain; VG, vegetable; FR, fruit; DA, dairy; PRO, protein source; FAT, healthy fats and oils; LEG, legume; and NUT, nut.

*Sodium values have been rounded to the nearest 5 mg.

DAY 2 AT 2,300 MG SODIUM	CALORIES	SODIUM (MG)*	FOOD GROUP
breakfast			
2 frozen blueberry waffles with	190	370	2 GR
¼ cup pancake syrup	100	55	
8 oz orange juice	110	0	2 FR
subtotal	**400**	**425**	
snack			
¼ cup seedless raisins	125	5	1 FR
2 oz dry-roasted peanuts, unsalted	340	0	1 NUT
subtotal	**465**	**5**	
lunch			
1 multigrain English muffin with	150	180	2 GR
⅔ cup *Curried Tuna Salad with Almonds* (page 222) or equal amount of very low sodium tuna	160	160	1 PRO
1 large apple	115	0	1 FR
8 oz fat-free milk	85	105	1 DA
subtotal	**510**	**445**	
snack			
8 oz low-sodium mixed-vegetable juice	80	140	2 VG
3 whole-grain crispbreads	60	95	1 GR
subtotal	**140**	**235**	
dinner			
restaurant take-out:			
⅔ cup beef and broccoli	130	710	1 VG, 1 PRO
½ cup mixed vegetables	35	260	1 VG
½ cup steamed plain rice	200	0	1 GR
½ cup mandarin oranges in juice	80	10	1 FR
12 oz green tea, unsweetened	0	0	
subtotal	**445**	**980**	
totals	**1,960**	**2,090**	**4 VG, 5 FR, 6 GR, 1 DA 2 PRO, 0 FAT, 1 NUT**

Note: GR indicates grain; VG, vegetable; FR, fruit; DA, dairy; PRO, protein source; FAT, healthy fats and oils; LEG, legume; and NUT, nut.

*Sodium values have been rounded to the nearest 5 mg.

DAY 3 AT 2,300 MG SODIUM	CALORIES	SODIUM (MG)*	FOOD GROUP
breakfast			
1 frozen low-calorie breakfast sandwich	210	480	1 GR, 1 PRO
8 oz fat-free milk	85	105	1 DA
1 medium banana	105	0	1 FR
subtotal	**400**	**585**	
snack			
1 oz almonds, unsalted	165	0	½ NUT
¼ cup dried apricots	100	0	1 FR
subtotal	**265**	**0**	
lunch			
2 oz whole-grain spaghetti	200	0	2 GR
½ cup spaghetti sauce	80	380	1 VG
2 tbsp shredded Parmesan cheese	45	150	½ DA
2 cups mixed salad greens	20	40	2 VG
2 tbsp low-fat oil and vinegar dressing	70	200	1 FAT
1 medium whole-wheat roll	100	170	1 GR
subtotal	**515**	**940**	
snack			
7 tortilla chips	140	120	1 GR
¼ cup salsa	20	260	½ VG
subtotal	**160**	**380**	
dinner			
3 oz *Pork Chops with Sage-Thyme Rub* (page 152)	160	190	1 PRO
1 cup sliced zucchini, cooked with	20	10	2 VG
2 tsp olive oil,	80	0	1 FAT
herbs, and 1⁄16 tsp salt	0	145	
1 cup cooked brown rice	225	10	2 GR
8 oz iced tea, unsweetened	0	0	
1 cup fat-free vanilla frozen yogurt	160	80	1 DA
subtotal	**645**	**435**	
totals	**1,985**	**2,340**	**5½ VG, 2 FR, 7 GR, 2½ DA, 2 PRO, 2 FAT, ½ NUT**

CHRISTY'S SECOND STEP-DOWN MENU PLAN AT 2,000 CALORIES AND 1,500 MG SODIUM

DAY 1 AT 1,500 MG SODIUM	CALORIES	SODIUM (MG)*	FOOD GROUP
breakfast			
1¼ cups shredded wheat minis with	170	0	2½ GR
8 oz fat-free milk	85	105	1 DA
½ cup blueberries	40	0	1 FR
1 medium banana, sliced	105	0	1 FR
subtotal	**400**	**105**	
snack			
3 tbsp low-sodium peanut butter	300	100	1½ NUT
3 whole-grain crispbreads	60	95	1 GR
subtotal	**360**	**195**	
lunch			
sandwich of			
2 slices low-sodium whole-grain bread with	140	200	2 GR
3 oz *Roasted Turkey* (page 160) or equal amount of plain chicken breast	135	45	1 PRO
½ cup chopped romaine and 3 slices tomato	10	5	1 VG
2 tsp honey mustard	20	50	
8 oz iced tea, unsweetened	0	0	
subtotal	**305**	**300**	
snack			
8 oz plain fat-free Greek yogurt with	120	85	1 DA
½ cup blueberries	40	0	1 FR
subtotal	**160**	**85**	

DAY 1 AT 1,500 MG SODIUM	CALORIES	SODIUM (MG)*	FOOD GROUP
dinner			
3 oz *Crunchy Oven-Fried Fish Fillets* (with *Cocktail Sauce*) (page 172) or equal size plain fish fillet	255	380	1 PRO
1 cup green beans, no-salt-added canned	40	20	2 VG
½ cup *Veggie Mac and Cheese* (page.192) or equal amount plain pasta with light tub margarine and herbs	100	160	1 GR
2 cups mixed salad greens	20	40	2 VG
2 tbsp *Thousand Island Dressing* (page 226)	35	115	1 FAT
4 oz white wine	100	5	
1 *Luscious Lemon Sponge Pudding* (page 248)	195	90	½ FR
subtotal	**745**	**810**	
totals	**1,970**	**1,495**	**5 VG, 3½ FR, 6½ GR, 2 DA, 2 PRO, 1 FAT, 1½ NUT**

Note: GR indicates grain; VG, vegetable; FR, fruit; DA, dairy; PRO, protein source; FAT, healthy fats and oils; LEG, legume; and NUT, nut.

*Sodium values have been rounded to the nearest 5 mg.

DAY 2 AT 1,500 MG SODIUM	CALORIES	SODIUM (MG)*	FOOD GROUP
breakfast			
2 *Pancakes with Blueberry-Vanilla Sauce* (page 238)	265	305	2 GR
8 oz orange juice	110	0	2 FR
subtotal	**375**	**305**	
snack			
¼ cup seedless raisins	125	5	1 FR
2 oz dry-roasted peanuts, unsalted	340	0	1 NUT
subtotal	**465**	**5**	
lunch			
1 multigrain English muffin with	150	180	2 GR
⅔ cup *Curried Tuna Salad with Almonds* (page 222) or equal amount of very low sodium tuna	160	160	1 PRO
1 large apple	115	0	1 FR
8 oz fat-free milk	85	105	1 DA
subtotal	**510**	**445**	
snack			
8 oz low-sodium mixed-vegetable juice	80	140	2 VG
½ cup carrot sticks	25	45	1 VG
subtotal	**105**	**185**	
dinner			
1½ cups *Beef-and-Broccoli Stir-Fry* (includes rice) (page 148)	310	560	2 VG, 1 GR, 1 PRO
½ cup mandarin oranges in juice with	80	10	1 FR
1 medium banana, sliced	105	0	1 FR
12 oz green tea, unsweetened	0	0	
subtotal	**495**	**570**	
totals	**1,950**	**1,510**	**5 VG, 6 FR, 5 GR, 1 DA, 2 PRO, 0 FAT, 1 NUT**

Note: GR indicates grain; VG, vegetable; FR, fruit; DA, dairy; PRO, protein source; FAT, healthy fats and oils; LEG, legume; and NUT, nut.

*Sodium values have been rounded to the nearest 5 mg.

DAY 3 AT 1,500 MG SODIUM	CALORIES	SODIUM (MG)*	FOOD GROUP
breakfast			
1 *Open-Face Breakfast Sandwich* (page 241)	165	295	1 GR, 1 PRO
8 oz fat-free milk	85	105	1 DA
1 medium banana	105	0	1 FR
subtotal	**355**	**400**	
snack			
1 oz almonds, unsalted	165	0	½ NUT
½ cup dried apricots	200	0	2 FR
subtotal	**365**	**0**	
lunch			
2 oz whole-grain spaghetti	200	0	2 GR
½ cup *Mamma Mia Marinara* (page 215)	55	15	1 VG
2 tbsp shredded Parmesan cheese	45	150	½ DA
2 cups mixed salad greens	20	40	2 VG
2 tbsp *Basil-Garlic Italian Dressing* (page 225)	85	145	1 FAT
1 medium whole-wheat roll	100	170	1 GR
subtotal	**505**	**520**	
snack			
¾ cup *Herbed Veggie Chips* (page 202)	110	205	1 VG
¼ cup *Fresh Tomato-Tomatillo Salsa* (page 210)	10	60	½ VG
subtotal	**120**	**265**	
dinner			
3 oz *Pork Chops with Sage-Thyme Rub* (page 152)	160	190	1 PRO
1 cup sliced zucchini cooked in	20	10	2 VG
2 tsp olive oil	80	0	1 FAT
herbs	0	0	
1 cup cooked brown rice	225	10	2 GR
1 cup fat-free vanilla frozen yogurt	160	80	1 DA
subtotal	**645**	**290**	
totals	**1,990**	**1,475**	**6½ VG, 3 FR, 6 GR, 2½ DA, 2 PRO, 2 FAT, ½ NUT**

PLANNING AHEAD WHEN EATING OUT

Thinking ahead also can save you lots of sodium when eating out. Because the same dish can vary wildly from restaurant to restaurant, try to obtain accurate information for the restaurant you'll be visiting and compare the options there. Compare this ordering plan for Owen, the salesman profiled in Chapter 3, with his meals on page 33, and you'll see that planning can make a difference.

OWEN'S ON-THE-ROAD ORDERING PLAN

ONE TYPICAL DAY'S CHOICES	CALORIES	SODIUM (MG)*	FOOD GROUP
breakfast			
"healthy" vegetable omelet with	300	690	1 VG, 1 PRO
½ cup fruit			1 FR
8 oz orange juice	110	0	2 FR
1 slice whole-wheat toast with	90	150	1 GR
2 tsp raspberry jam	50	0	
8 oz fat-free milk	85	105	1 DA
subtotal	**635**	**945**	
lunch			
apple chicken salad, full order	500	830	2 VG, 1 PRO, 1 FR
subtotal	**500**	**830**	
snack			
1 protein bar	240	200	1 GR
1 large apple	115	0	1 FR
8 oz plain fat-free Greek yogurt	120	85	1 DA
subtotal	**475**	**285**	
dinner			
3 oz plain grilled salmon fillet with	660	610	1 PRO
1 cup mixed broccoli and rice			1 VG, 1 GR
1 slice French bread	80	160	1 GR
2 x 4 oz white wine	200	10	
subtotal	**940**	**780**	
totals	**2,550**	**2,840**	**4 VG, 5 FR, 4 GR, 2 DA, 3 PRO, 0 FAT**

Note: GR indicates grain; VG, vegetable; FR, fruit; DA, dairy; PRO, protein source; FAT, healthy fats and oils; LEG, legume; and NUT, nut.

***Sodium values have been rounded to the nearest 5 mg.**

GETTING CREATIVE IN THE KITCHEN

One of the joys of planning your menus is being able to choose what to prepare. Cooking at home can be creative and fun—and it can allow you to serve delicious, lower-sodium meals that will be kind to your heart. Contrary to conventional wisdom, eating less salt does not have to mean enjoying food less. In fact, many people say that they taste a wider range of different flavors once they put aside the salt and its one-note taste.

Season for Flavor

When you get past the idea that salt is needed to bring out the flavor of food, you'll find a new world of taste possibilities. Think fresh and intense and experiment with all the delicious ways to replace salt while adding depth and interest to your dishes. For some new tastes, try some of the ideas in "Sodium-Free Flavoring Suggestions" in the Toolkit (Part IV, page 264).

GO FRESH

- Use fresh herbs when possible. In most cases, they give more vibrant flavor than dried. For a brighter taste, add them at the last minute.
- Grind whole spices as you need them. They'll be fresher and provide the most powerful flavor impact.
- Buy only small amounts of dried herbs and the spices that you purchase preground so they won't lose their punch. The more often you rotate your supply, the more intense the flavors will be.
- Add hot chiles to your dishes for a little bite. Peppers from the produce aisle are very low in sodium and have a lot more flavor than pickled peppers, which are high in sodium.
- Buy fresh gingerroot and freeze it in peeled chunks so you'll always have some on hand for its zingy flavor. Grate gingerroot using a ginger grater, rasp grater, or flat, sheet-type grater.
- Squeeze citrus juice on foods to enhance flavor. Wonderful on fish, citrus also works well on many vegetables, such as broccoli and green beans. Try different vinegars too, especially on greens.
- Perk up flavor with citrus zest, the part of the peel without the bitter white pith. Grate the peel or use a vegetable peeler to remove wide slices, which you can cut into thin strips.

INTENSIFY

- Use dried mushrooms, tomatoes, chiles, cherries, cranberries, and currants to impart a more intense flavor than the fresh versions. If you reconstitute these foods by soaking them, use any leftover "broth" to enrich other dishes.
- Dry-roast seeds, nuts, and whole spices to bring out their full flavor.
- Reduce liquids such as wines and broths to deepen and intensify their flavors. (Avoid cooking wines, which are high in sodium.)
- Marinate meats in low-sodium mixtures for rich, layered flavor without added salt or sodium-laden sauces. Marinating also helps tenderize tougher cuts of meat, so consider using a homemade version, such as Spicy-Sweet Citrus-Cilantro Marinade (page 214) instead of high-sodium commercial marinades or tenderizers.
- Refrigerate drippings from roasted meat or poultry to allow the fat to rise to the top and harden. Once you've discarded the fat, use the rich liquid to intensify the flavor of stews, sauces, and soups.
- Cook foods wrapped in aluminum foil or parchment paper to seal in delicious natural juices.

REPLACE

- Replace flavored salts, such as garlic and onion, with the comparable powders. You'll get just as much flavor but with zero sodium.
- Fill a salt or pepper shaker with a combination of crumbled dried herbs and finely ground spices to use at the table instead of salt, or buy salt-free herb blends.
- Instead of using high-sodium bottled mustard, try using dry mustard mixed with water.
- Wrap foods in lettuce or cabbage leaves instead of in high-sodium breads or flour tortillas.
- Make your own low-sodium salad dressings (see pages 224–226 for recipes). For the convenience of commercial bottled dressings, prepare a double batch or more, depending on how long the dressing will keep in the refrigerator.
- Control sodium by making your own versions of common sauces (see page 206) and favorite condiments.

SALT SUBSTITUTES If you're considering buying a salt substitute, be sure to read the labels. Many salt substitutes contain a large amount of potassium and very little sodium; most people can use them freely, but not people who have certain health conditions (kidney disease, for example) or take medications that cause the body to retain potassium. Talk with your healthcare professional about whether a salt substitute is a good option for you.

Shop and Cook Heart-Smart

When you're cooking at home, you are in control. Stick to these basic heart-healthy cooking techniques to keep sodium, calories, and unhealthy fats at a minimum.

- Always use the lowest-sodium products available. These may be labeled "sodium-free," "salt-free," "no-salt-added," "very low sodium," or "low-sodium." The difference between these products and their "regular" counterparts can be significant, so be sure to compare nutrition facts panels.
- Check regularly for newly introduced products. Read nutrition facts labels often, since newer products may be low in sodium without advertising that benefit on the front of the packaging.
- Use a nonstick skillet so you can cook foods with a minimum of oil, or use cooking spray. (Check the warranty information from your cookware's manufacturer. Some caution against using cooking spray on nonstick surfaces.)
- Trim away and discard all visible fat before cooking meat. For poultry, remove the fat and skin except when roasting whole poultry; in that case, discard the cooked skin before eating the poultry. Raw skin will be easier to remove if you use paper towels or a clean cloth to take hold of it. To help prevent the spread of bacteria, scrub the cutting surface and utensils well with hot, sudsy water after preparing meat or poultry.
- Bump up your intake of vegetables and fruits by using them in unexpected ways. Add chopped spinach to lasagna, include shredded zucchini in meat loaf, put pumpkin purée in pancake batter, and toss some berries or peeled orange wedges into your salads. Be creative!
- Stretch the amount of ground poultry or meat you have by adding chopped vegetables to feed more people and incorporate more veggies.

For more ideas and delicious ways to shop and cook heart-smart, check out the more than 60 lower-sodium recipes found throughout Part III, "Sodium Sense by Food Type—with Recipes."

CHAPTER 9

Healthy Sodium for Life

The previous chapters in this section have focused on specific strategies you can use to lower the amount of sodium in your diet, but these strategies can have a long-term impact only if you turn them into lasting habits. By trying out various strategies in the context of your own life, you can find out which ones work for you. Now it's time to step back, look at the big picture, and see how to integrate a lower-sodium, balanced diet with the other important lifestyle changes that lead to a longer, healthier life.

HEALTHY LIFESTYLE STRATEGIES

✓ Apply eating strategies to reduce sodium in your diet.
✓ Monitor your blood pressure regularly.
✓ Establish a regular routine of physical activity to keep blood pressure and weight in check.
✓ Manage stress to protect your heart.
✓ Avoid smoking and excessive alcohol use.
✓ Stay motivated to maintain healthy habits for life.

EATING STRATEGIES FOR LONG-TERM HEALTH

After focusing on the "how" of cutting back on sodium, you can put the numbers into perspective by remembering the "why." The primary reason to reduce sodium is to prevent an increase in blood pressure, which can damage your health, especially your cardiovascular health. With that aim in mind, here's a recap of the ways you can make the transition to a lower-sodium lifestyle.

- **EDUCATE YOURSELF:** Learn where sodium lurks and assess how much you are actually consuming.
- **START WITH SMALL CHANGES:** To jump-start your transition, find the easiest ways to *rethink*, *replace*, and *reduce* the highest-sodium foods you eat often.
- **TARGET HIGH-SODIUM FOODS AT HOME:** *Rethink, replace,* and *reduce* the high-sodium foods you bring into your own kitchen.
- **IDENTIFY HIGH-SODIUM FOODS WHEN EATING OUT:** *Rethink, replace,* and *reduce* the high-sodium foods you choose when you eat out.
- **STAY FOCUSED ON EATING WELL:** Follow the American Heart Association diet and lifestyle recommendations on how to achieve a balanced, nutritious diet.
- **PLAN AHEAD WITH LOWER-SODIUM MENUS:** Create your own lower-sodium eating plan that incorporates your favorite healthy recipes and meets your scheduling needs.

Each approach provides a set of actions you can take to cut back on sodium. Each action alone will help get you closer to your goal of a lower-sodium diet; but even better, the actions *together* will greatly increase your odds of significantly reducing your sodium consumption and improving your health in the future.

Assess Your Successes

After several weeks of applying the sodium-cutting strategies, take some time to evaluate how your efforts are paying off. Spend a week or two tracking your sodium intake, just as you did at the beginning of this process. (You can find a blank tracker template in the Toolkit, Part IV, page 254.) Once you've gathered enough data to reflect your typical eating habits now, compare the current daily average with the baseline results from your original tracker. In addition to determining whether you have been successful in cutting back on your total amount of sodium, you may also be able to identify patterns that will reinforce your understanding of which strategies work best for you and why.

Check Your Blood Pressure

Have your blood pressure measured after you have actively been cutting back on the sodium in your diet for several weeks. If you find that your blood pressure has dropped, you know that your body is reacting positively to the changes you have made. If it hasn't dropped, however, don't feel that you haven't benefited. Not everyone is immediately affected by a lowered sodium intake, and the cumulative effects of eating too much sodium can take a long time to show themselves. Remember that blood pressure is affected by several powerful factors in addition to sodium intake (for more details, see Chapter 2). Whatever else your body is experiencing, you are helping protect your cardiovascular system by not adding excess salt to it. To continue to track the effects of your lower-sodium diet, monitor your blood pressure regularly. Most healthy people should have blood pressure checks at least once every two years.

HEALTHY LIFESTYLE, HEALTHY BLOOD PRESSURE

Living a healthy lifestyle is the best way to keep your blood pressure low and protect your heart and overall well-being. Eating a nutritious diet—which includes cutting back on sodium—is an essential part of that healthy lifestyle, but other factors are important, too. Participating in regular physical activity, maintaining a healthy weight, managing stress, avoiding smoking, and limiting alcohol are key components.

Add Regular Physical Activity to Your Routine

Regular physical activity offers so many health benefits that you simply can't afford to put off being more active. (Congratulations if you're already on an appropriate exercise regimen!) Adding exercise to your daily routine will increase both the length and the quality of your life, and being more active on a regular basis has both physical and mental benefits. In addition to building strength and toning your body, you'll feel improvements in your general well-being over time.

Your body benefits because exercise:

- Increases your blood circulation and improves delivery of oxygen and nutrients to your body's cells
- Helps develop your endurance, strength, and flexibility
- Burns calories to help keep your weight at a healthy level
- Enhances your immune system
- Helps maintain bone density
- Improves quality of sleep

Your mind benefits because exercise:

- Increases the flow of oxygen to the brain, which can improve your mental acuity and memory
- Releases tension and counteracts the negative effects of stress
- Relieves anxiety, depression, and anger

These benefits result in tangible, long-term rewards, such as:

- Lowered blood pressure
- Reduced blood cholesterol
- Decreased risk of heart disease, stroke, and diabetes
- More energy and a more optimistic outlook

Participating in physical activities becomes even more important as you get older. For example, if you are middle-aged, regular exercise can help counteract the metabolic changes that come with aging. Aerobic conditioning combined with resistance training will help you reduce arterial stiffening, maintain muscle mass, and lessen bone loss as you age. Recent studies have suggested that regular physical activity can even help slow the progression of existing heart disease no matter what your age.

AVOID THE DANGERS OF BEING INACTIVE If knowing the established benefits of physical activity isn't enough to get you moving, consider the harmful effects of sitting still. The disease risk of physical *in*activity is roughly equivalent to that of having high blood pressure, having high cholesterol, or smoking! In fact, living an inactive life can be considered as dangerous to your health as smoking a pack of cigarettes a day.

Without regular physical exercise, your body will lose its strength, stamina, and ability to function well. Like your other muscles, your heart needs to work on a regular basis to stay in good condition. Aerobic activities, such as running and dancing, keep your heart strong so it can pump oxygen-rich blood effectively. If you aren't exercising, your heart isn't getting the workout it needs to stay in good condition and to deliver blood at a lower heart rate and at lower pressure.

Another result of being inactive is that you have a greater likelihood of being obese or overweight. On the other hand, physical activity burns calories and therefore helps you keep your weight in check. If you're eating more calories than you're using, you will gradually gain unwanted pounds; as you get older, you need fewer calories, making it even harder to manage your weight if you aren't exercising and burning energy. Added weight can raise blood pressure and increase the chance that you'll develop diabetes.

AMP UP YOUR ACTIVITY LEVEL Almost 70 percent of Americans aren't getting the amount of exercise they need to be healthy, but you don't have to be part of that group. If you're sedentary now, take the time to schedule in some activities that will get your heart pumping. If you're already enjoying a workout routine, find ways to bump it up a notch or add another type of activity. Either way, you have lots of fun options to choose from, ranging from gentle activities to extreme workouts. If you don't think you'd enjoy joining a gym or jogging through the neighborhood, try some different things until you find what is most appealing to and appropriate for you. Some possibilities include:

- Aerobic dance
- Bowling
- Golfing
- Bicycling
- Swimming and water aerobics
- Softball, basketball, flag football, soccer, and tennis
- Jumping rope
- Hiking and walking
- Mowing and gardening
- Boot camp
- Kickboxing

When adding physical activity to your routine, remember that it is the regularity, not the intensity, with which you exercise that provides the lasting health benefits. Even 10 minutes a day will get you started toward a healthier lifestyle. As you work toward the recommended goals, you can add physical activity in increments, as long as each session lasts at least 10 minutes. The key to success is to find something you can enjoy so you'll make regular exercise a permanent part of your lifestyle.

Your weekly target is to include sessions of aerobic activity that add up to:

- *150 minutes of moderate intensity.* At this level, your heart rate increases but you can still talk.

or

- *75 minutes of vigorous intensity.* At this level, your heart rate increases significantly, you breathe rapidly, and you can say only a few words without needing to catch your breath.

or

- An equivalent combination of the two.

For some ideas on how to reach these goals, try different combinations of activity and intensity. For example, you could walk briskly for 30 minutes on five days (moderate intensity) or take a 60-minute step aerobics class twice a week and walk for 30 minutes on the weekend. (You need to spend roughly twice as long exercising at moderate intensity as at vigorous intensity.)

Maintain a Healthy Weight

If you're concerned enough about your health to cut back on sodium, you should also take steps to be sure you maintain a weight that is healthy for your height. Statistics show that overweight and obese people are much more likely to have high blood pressure, a major risk factor for cardiovascular disease. Being overweight can also contribute to the risk for other health problems. To carry extra weight, your body needs more energy. To provide that energy, your heart must pump harder, increasing blood pressure and the stress on your circulatory system. Over time, the heavier workload can cause your heart to enlarge and weaken.

If you're overweight, losing as little as 10 percent of your body weight can help reduce your blood pressure or prevent it from rising to dangerous levels. Managing your weight can also help maintain healthy blood cholesterol and prevent diabetes. To lose extra pounds, you must reduce your calorie intake and add enough physical activity so that you burn more energy than you take in. For an effective weight-loss program, you need to know your recommended calorie intake. Compare that with the number of calories you are actually eating and the number of calories you are burning through physical activity to see how much you need to cut back. (For more information on determining your calorie intake and healthy weight loss, visit www.heart.org.) As you work toward cutting calories, be sure that you also continue to include the same nutritious foods detailed in Chapter 7, "Stay Focused on Eating Well," such as fruits and vegetables, almost all of which are low in calories, and fiber-rich whole grains, which can help you feel full.

Your goal is to lose weight slowly and safely so you can *keep* the pounds off. To do that, it's best to aim for a gradual weight loss of one to two pounds per week. Simple and effective techniques to lose weight include adding a routine of aerobic physical activity, eating smaller portions, substituting lower-calorie foods for high-calorie ones, following a safe and healthy weight-loss diet plan, or combining all these options. Talk with your healthcare provider to decide which approach is best for you.

Manage Stress and Avoid Harmful Habits

For most people, stress is a reality of life. In today's fast-paced environment, just keeping up with life's demands can lead to nonstop overload. Many of us react by turning to unhealthy habits that bring temporary relief but have harmful consequences. Eating unhealthy foods and/or overeating, smoking, and drinking too much alcohol, for example, all increase the risk for high blood pressure and therefore the risk for heart attack and stroke.

LEARN HOW TO COPE WITH STRESS Although a direct connection between stress and heart disease has not been scientifically confirmed, researchers are studying how stress affects heart health—specifically blood pressure. When you feel stressed, your body reacts by releasing two hormones, adrenaline and cortisol, into the bloodstream. These hormones make your heart beat faster and constrict blood vessels so your body will be ready for "fight or flight"; these responses cause a temporary increase in blood pressure that goes away when the stressful situation is over. Fight or flight was an effective defense mechanism for our ancestors, but in today's world, we are constantly confronted by stresses that we can't deal with by fighting or taking flight. When the stress reaction continues for longer periods than our bodies are equipped to handle, we suffer both physical and mental consequences. Being in a state of chronic stress puts more strain on your circulatory system and compromises your feeling of well-being.

To counteract these negatives, it's important to learn effective techniques to cope with the stress in your life. You can better control your body's responses by being mindful of what difficulties you face routinely, what is within your power to change, and how you can best make those changes.

To get started, try these stress-reducing suggestions:

- Engage in some form of physical activity on a regular basis.
- Give yourself enough time to get things done and avoid procrastinating.
- Don't overschedule and do learn to say no.
- Recognize when you have no control in a situation and try to accept what you can't change.
- Know your stress triggers and find ways to avoid them.
- Nurture supportive relationships and talk over your problems with friends and family.
- Set aside time to sit quietly, breathe deeply, and let your mind wander.
- Pursue the things that bring you pleasure and try not to hurry through life.

QUIT SMOKING AND AVOID SECONDHAND SMOKE There is no doubt that smoking and exposing yourself to secondhand smoke put you at much greater risk for heart disease, stroke, and other dangerous illnesses. When you inhale smoke, you breathe in chemicals that cause your arteries to narrow, which reduces blood flow, makes your heart work harder, and increases blood pressure. Smoking also decreases your ability to exercise and increases the tendency of blood to clot.

Smoking is the number one cause of premature death in the United States. A smoker's risk of dying from heart disease is two to three times that of a nonsmoker. If you smoke now, find a way to quit. Let your health-care provider help you identify an approach, such as counseling or nicotine replacement, that will enable you to quit for good. If you need help, enlist your family and friends, go online, and turn to support groups and the many other resources available. Regardless of how long you have been a smoker, your risk of heart disease and stroke will begin to drop dramatically as soon as you stop smoking.

LIMIT YOUR USE OF ALCOHOL Although some studies have shown that drinking moderate amounts of alcohol results in health benefits, research also consistently shows that people who drink more than moderate levels tend to develop high blood pressure. Alcohol is a major source of calories and can contribute to weight gain, which in turn can further increase blood pressure. A moderate amount means no more than two drinks per day for a man and no more than one drink per day for a woman. One drink is 12 ounces of beer, 5 ounces of wine, or 1½ ounces of 80-proof liquor. If you don't drink alcohol now, don't start; if you drink more than is considered moderate, find ways to cut back.

MAINTAINING MOTIVATION

To stay motivated and engaged, think positively and consider all the things you are doing to be healthier and stronger. Remember that you have choices. By adopting a lower-sodium lifestyle, you are making your health a top priority, even if doing so seems challenging at first. Changing well-established habits takes effort and resolve. Balancing the different aspects of your life—work, social schedules, family needs, economic realities, and health considerations—can leave you feeling pulled in many directions at once. Your situation is unique, of course, and only you can decide which strategies will work and what rewards will keep you motivated. Remember that it takes repetition for a new behavior to become habit, so be vigilant about continuing to choose healthy behaviors. When you find the right combination of strategies—*rethink, replace,* and *reduce*—you'll be able to establish healthier habits today that will last the rest of your life.

Savor New Tastes and Tackle Old Challenges

After a few weeks of concentrating on managing your sodium intake, you will find the task easier and more automatic. By then, your taste buds should be better adjusted to foods that are less salty, and you—like smokers who discover a whole new world of taste and smell when they quit—should be able to really appreciate the full spectrum of flavors in what you eat and drink.

It can, however, be hard to maintain enthusiasm when the initial excitement of tackling a new resolution wears off. That's when you may be most tempted to return to some, if not all, of your high-sodium habits. To combat the temptation to be less vigilant and to keep your commitment top of mind, pay extra attention to your dietary "danger zones" and how they influence your choices. For example, if you know you tend to turn to unhealthy comfort foods when you're under stress, choose an alternate behavior you can substitute—*before* things get so hectic that you can't think clearly enough to make a smart decision. Perhaps you travel often and you know that healthy food options are very limited at the airport. Plan to pack a few healthy snacks, such as portable fruit, instead of relying on the fast food you usually buy in such situations. Whatever your own potential downfalls may be, try to identify them and find a solution before they can derail you.

When the urge to "cheat" threatens your commitment to go lower-sodium or when you are stressed, employ a coping technique that will give you the upper hand. Keep temptations at a distance, occupy yourself with a distraction, or replace an unhealthy habit with a good one. For example:

- Don't bring high-sodium foods into your house—or at least keep them out of easy reach. If a particular food will be hard to resist, make it difficult to get in the first place.
- Keep your hands busy. Find something else to do with them besides eat. Keep the daily crossword puzzle handy, turn your attention to minor chores, or distract yourself by picking up the phone to call or text friends or family.
- Prepare healthy snacks to replace vending-machine choices, and keep them on hand at work and at home. Try dipping celery sticks, strips of bell pepper, and cauliflower or broccoli florets in homemade hummus

(recipe on page 204) or noshing on Hot Soft Pretzels (page 196), Herbed Veggie Chips (page 202), or Nutty Cereal-and-Seeds Snack Mix (page 205).

If once in a while you crave a super-salty snack or feel so stressed that you turn to a food you've been avoiding, it's okay. Just remember your original reasons for wanting to lower your sodium intake and to eat healthy. Remind yourself to take life one day at a time and not to be discouraged: it's always better to do something that gets you closer to your goal than to do nothing at all.

Celebrate Your Successes

Since you began the process of changing your diet, what steps have worked for you? Did your follow-up tracker show a reduction in sodium? Did your blood pressure go down? Be sure to congratulate—and reward—yourself for each and every one of your successes! For every move you make toward lowering the sodium in your diet, give yourself something that makes you feel good. Decide in advance on a treat that will motivate you—perhaps a new book, a massage, or a gift card to your favorite store. Whatever reward you choose, find one that is both enjoyable and healthy. You might want to go to the movies, but you'll need to stay away from the popcorn and other high-sodium concessions. Instead, why not consider renting a movie and treating yourself to Three-Way Popcorn (page 198) at home.

Ultimately, the real reward for sticking to your commitment will be a longer, more vital life. Perhaps you're a parent who wants to provide a healthy diet for your young children, or a busy executive who wants to stay in top form, or maybe you're middle-aged and facing a diagnosis of high blood pressure or heart disease. No matter who you are or why you want to cut back on sodium, doing so will significantly increase your chances of avoiding a debilitating or deadly disease later in life. When you combine those better odds with the benefits of a healthy lifestyle, your choices will have a profoundly positive effect on your overall well-being.

PART III

Sodium Sense by Food Type—with Recipes

More than 40 percent of the sodium in the average American diet comes from just a few types of food, according to recent findings from the CDC. In fact, as shown below in the list of the top sodium sources, we collectively eat so much of certain types of food that it's important to understand how each category contributes to our total sodium intake.

TOP 10 SOURCES OF SODIUM

1. Breads and rolls
2. Cold cuts and cured meats, such as deli or packaged ham and turkey
3. Pizza
4. Fresh and processed chicken and turkey
5. Soups
6. Sandwiches, including burgers
7. Cheese
8. Pasta dishes with sauce
9. Mixed meat dishes, such as meat loaf with sauce
10. Snacks, such as chips, pretzels, and popcorn

All of the foods on the top 10 list have been processed in some way, which accounts for the added sodium they contain, since most foods in their natural state contain very little sodium. However, not all manufactured foods are created equally and not all processed foods should be considered completely unhealthy just because they contain sodium; many are enriched and fortified with important minerals and vitamins. When making your own food decisions, remember to weigh not only how much sodium is in a product but also the overall health benefits it has to offer and how often you include it in your diet.

The information in the following sections is broken down by food type. For each food category, you'll find sodium values for some typical foods that are widely available in grocery stores. Given the thousands of food products on the market, these values reflect a representative sampling only and do not necessarily reflect the lowest or highest sodium values available for a particular food. (The values have been rounded to the nearest multiple of 5 mg to make it easier to compare similar products, such as ketchup and no-salt-added ketchup.) We've listed many of the recipes (with page cross-references) in this book along with their sodium values as another point of comparison to grocery store products. When comparing the sodium values in the charts, be sure to take note of the serving sizes.

Here you'll also find tips and useful information to help you become more aware of hidden sodium and make better choices among products. Finally, you'll find more than 60 recipes designated by section. Each recipe is a lower-sodium alternative to a typically high-sodium food, such as chicken nuggets, ranch salad dressing, or broccoli-cheese soup, and each will show you how to knock out most of the sodium while keeping in the flavor.

BREADS AND GRAINS

One of the biggest contributors to Americans' intake of sodium is bread. Salt helps control the dough's rising process and is also used as a preservative to keep bread products fresh longer; salt adds flavor, especially to white breads, which have been so refined that they have been stripped not only of their nutrients but also of their taste. Grains themselves are low in sodium, but so many favorite preparations involve salty sauces, seasonings, and cheese that most pasta and rice dishes contain a surprisingly high amount of sodium. Whole-grain breads and grain products are an important part of a fiber-rich diet, however, so it's important to include them in your meal plans. Just be sure to read the nutrition facts panels and choose the products that are lower in sodium.

TRY THESE LOWER-SODIUM BREAD AND GRAIN RECIPES:

- Pizza Dough (page 135) with Margherita Topping (page 137)
- Whole-Grain and Honey Bread (page 138)
- Corn Bread Dressing (page 140)
- Zucchini Quick Bread with Nuts and Fruit (page 142)
- Fried Rice (page 143)

SPOTLIGHT ON: Pizza An American favorite, pizza comes in number three on the CDC's list of the top 10 sources of sodium in the average person's diet in the United States. Sodium is found in the crust, the sauce, the cheese, and some of the toppings, and the total can easily add up to a day's worth of sodium, if not more. To enjoy pizza without all the sodium, try making your own dough; it's not as difficult as you might think and it freezes well. (See the recipe on page 135.) Look for lower-sodium sauces (or make your own with the recipe on page 215) and cheeses, and top the pizza with roasted veggies instead of sodium-laden processed meats, such as pepperoni.

SODIUM IN SELECTED BREADS AND GRAINS

FOOD	SODIUM (MG)*
corn bread mix, 1 oz	230–455
Corn Bread (page 141), 1 piece	90
quick-bread mix, 1 oz	285–365
Zucchini Quick Bread with Nuts and Fruit (page 142), 1 slice	110
bread crumbs, seasoned, ¼ cup	530–560
bread crumbs, plain, ¼ cup	200–220
panko, seasoned, ¼ cup	135–430
panko, plain, ¼ cup	20–45
bagel, plain, 3.5 oz	520–600
bagel, plain, thin, 1.5 oz	240–250
English muffin, whole-wheat	200–265
pita bread, whole-wheat, 6-inch	320–340
whole-wheat bread, 1 slice	130–160
whole-wheat bread, 1 slice, thin	95
Whole-Grain and Honey Bread (page 138), 1 slice	50
white bread, 1 slice	130–135
whole-wheat sourdough bread, 1 slice	150
flour tortillas, 6-inch	140–190
corn tortillas, 6-inch	5–35
cheese pizza, frozen, ⅛ of 12-inch	405–640
pepperoni pizza, frozen, ⅛ of 12-inch	370–685
Pizza Dough with Margherita Topping (page 135), 1 slice	150
whole-wheat pasta, any variety, 1 oz	0
brown rice, ready to heat, ½ cup	5–50
brown rice, instant, 1 oz	0–10
rice mix, pilaf, 1 oz	320–470
rice mix, Mexican, 1 oz	315–390
rice mix, Cajun, 1 oz	270–345
fried rice mix, 1 oz	290–625
Fried Rice (page 143), ½ cup	200

***Sodium values have been rounded to the nearest 5 mg.**

SODIUM-SAVING SOLUTIONS

- All processed breads contain sodium because salt is needed to manufacture them. However, some breads are lower in sodium than others. Be sure to choose whole-grain varieties, such as whole-wheat; a whole grain should be the first ingredient listed.
- Look for thin sandwich buns or bread slices; both options help you limit your sodium.
- To reduce the sodium (and calories) in your favorite bagel, hollow out some of the bread and fill the well with a low-sodium nut butter, or try our Curried Tuna Salad with Almonds (page 222). Also, look for the thin varieties for a big sodium savings.
- When shopping for tortillas, pita breads, and sandwich wraps, take notice of the different sizes. You can reduce your sodium intake if you choose the ones with smaller diameters.
- When shopping for flour or cornmeal, avoid the self-rising varieties. There is a huge difference in the amount of sodium compared to regular flour types: self-rising flour has 155 mg of sodium per cup, and all-purpose flour has only 3 mg; 1 cup of regular yellow cornmeal has about 4 mg of sodium compared to 1,860 mg in self-rising cornmeal.
- Sandwiches can be loaded with sodium, especially those you buy when eating out. For starters, just the two slices of bread will, on average, contribute about 300 mg of sodium. Add the salty sandwich fillings, such as cheese and processed meat, and the condiments, such as mustard and pickle slices, and you have sodium overload.
- If you like to bring sandwiches to work or include them in your children's school lunch boxes, think beyond high-sodium fillings. Consider roasting a turkey (see recipe on page 160) on the weekend and using slices of it for sandwiches during the week; this will save you on sodium, even if you usually buy lower-sodium processed turkey. What about having tuna salad (see recipe on page 222) topped with dark green leafy lettuce and a slice of red onion, or low-sodium peanut butter and slices of banana? A veggie option is filling your sandwiches with slightly mashed avocado and slices of tomato and red onion, topped with cilantro leaves.
- Sandwiches often include high-sodium condiments, such as mayonnaise, mustard, and ketchup, so be mindful of how much you use. (See "Sauces, Gravies, Condiments, and Seasonings.") To use less of the

salty condiments but still get plenty of flavor, experiment with "stretching" them with healthier options; for instance, make the mayo go further by mixing in green onions or herbs, such as dill or basil, or adding minced fresh jalapeños or roasted red bell peppers.

- If you like a pickle and chips with your sandwich, you'll be adding a lot of sodium to your meal. Consider eating a lower-sodium sandwich, cutting down on the portion size of the sides, or finding lower-sodium alternatives. For example, instead of eating a whole pickle, try just a wedge or buy sandwich slices and use only a few pieces. Either choice will lower the sodium level.
- Instead of having a traditional sandwich with two slices of bread, try a whole-grain pita pocket or wrap the filling in a Bibb lettuce leaf. Either choice will cut the sodium considerably.
- Is Friday pizza day at work? An individual, or personal-size, pizza can send your sodium levels through the roof. You can consume about 1,000 mg just from the crust served by many national pizza chains. Cut that number by choosing the thin crust (whole-wheat, if it's available) and avoiding the deep-dish crust.
- Look for unseasoned instant brown rice or frozen brown rice that is low in sodium. Both take almost no time to cook and provide whole-grain goodness. To impart more flavor or add texture, cook the instant rice in low-sodium broth or sprinkle either kind of rice with herbs, chopped green onions, or chopped unsalted nuts before serving.
- Grains and pastas packaged with sauce or seasoning packets, such as rice mixes, ramen noodles, stuffing, and macaroni and cheese, are usually high in sodium. Read nutrition facts panels carefully because there are *huge* variations in sodium levels among these products.
- Avoid putting salt in the water when preparing pasta and rice. If you want to impart flavor to the water, add dried Italian seasoning, other herbs or salt-free blends, a squeeze of fresh lemon juice, or a bay leaf (be sure to remove the bay leaf before serving the food).
- Like other foods made with refined flour, white pasta is low in nutrition and bland in flavor, which is often why salt is added to the cooking water or salty sauces are eaten with it. Whole-grain pasta, on the other hand, is much more nutritious and has more flavor.

Pizza Dough

This recipe makes enough dough for *two* 12-inch crisp-thin pizzas. You can bake both of them or freeze half the dough to bake another day. We've included a fragrant tomato-and-basil-based topping for one crust (see page 137), or create one of your own, using fresh ingredients for flavor rather than the usual high-sodium items such as pepperoni, sausage, and anchovies.

SERVES 16
1 slice per serving

- 1 cup lukewarm water (105°F to 115°F)
- 1 teaspoon active dry yeast
- 1½ cups all-purpose flour, 3 to 4 tablespoons all-purpose flour, and ¼ cup all-purpose flour, divided use
- 1 cup cake flour
- ¼ cup toasted wheat germ
- ¼ teaspoon salt
- Cooking spray
- 2 teaspoons cornmeal
- Margherita Topping (optional; recipe follows)

1. In a small bowl, combine the water and yeast, stirring to dissolve. Let stand for 5 minutes.

2. Meanwhile, in a large bowl, stir together 1½ cups all-purpose flour, the cake flour, wheat germ, and salt.

3. When the yeast is ready, add it to the flour mixture, stirring until the dough starts to pull away from the side of the bowl.

4. Using the 3 to 4 tablespoons all-purpose flour, lightly flour a flat surface. Turn out the dough. Knead for 6 to 7 minutes, gradually adding, if needed, enough of the remaining ¼ cup all-purpose flour to make the dough smooth and elastic. (The dough shouldn't be dry or stick to the surface. You may not need any of the additional ¼ cup all-purpose flour, or you may need the entire amount if the dough is too sticky.)

5. Using cooking spray, lightly spray a large bowl and a piece of plastic wrap large enough to cover the top of the bowl. Transfer the dough to the bowl, turning to coat all sides with the cooking spray. Cover the bowl with the plastic

CONTINUED

wrap with the sprayed side down. Let the dough rise in a warm, draft-free place (about 85°F) for about 2 hours, or until doubled in bulk.

6. Preheat the oven to 450°F. Depending on how many crusts you are baking, lightly sprinkle one or two pizza pans or large baking sheets with the cornmeal. Set aside.

7. Punch the dough down. Divide it in half. Using a small amount of all-purpose flour, lightly flour a flat surface. Roll each half you are baking now into a 12-inch circle. Transfer to the pan(s). Top with Margherita Topping or as desired.

8. Bake for 12 to 15 minutes, or until the crust is golden brown and the topping is heated through.

9. To freeze the pizza dough for later use, follow the preceding directions until you have divided the dough in half (skip step 6). Lightly spray a resealable freezer bag or bags with cooking spray. Put the dough in and seal tightly. Freeze the dough for up to three months. Before baking, let the dough thaw in the refrigerator for at least 8 hours. Let the dough come to room temperature, 1 to 2 hours, before rolling it out and making the pizza as directed.

PER SERVING

PIZZA DOUGH

Calories 83
Total Fat 0.5 g
  Saturated Fat 0.0 g
  Trans Fat 0.0 g
  Polyunsaturated Fat 0.0 g
  Monounsaturated Fat 0.0 g
Cholesterol 0 mg
Sodium 37 mg

Carbohydrates 17 g
  Fiber 1 g
  Sugars 0 g
Protein 3 g
Calcium 4 mg
Potassium 41 mg
Dietary Exchanges:
1 starch

Margherita Topping

SERVES 8

enough for one 12-inch pizza

1 14.5-ounce can no-salt-added diced tomatoes, well drained

2 teaspoons olive oil

½ teaspoon dried oregano, crumbled

¼ teaspoon pepper

⅛ teaspoon salt

½ cup shredded low-fat mozzarella cheese

½ cup fresh basil, coarsely chopped

2 tablespoons shredded or grated Parmesan cheese

1. In a small bowl, stir together the tomatoes, oil, oregano, and pepper. Spread over the pizza crust.

2. Sprinkle with the salt. Top, in order, with the mozzarella, basil, and Parmesan.

3. Bake as directed in the preceding recipe.

SODIUM SMARTS: If you can't imagine eating pizza without pepperoni, think of it as a garnish rather than as a topping: cut up one round and sprinkle the pieces over one slice of pizza.

PER SERVING

PIZZA DOUGH WITH MARGHERITA TOPPING

Calories 124
Total Fat 2.5 g
Saturated Fat 0.5 g
Trans Fat 0.0 g
Polyunsaturated Fat 0.5 g
Monounsaturated Fat 1.0 g
Cholesterol 3 mg
Sodium 151 mg
Carbohydrates 20 g
Fiber 2 g
Sugars 2 g
Protein 5 g
Calcium 97 mg
Potassium 176 mg
Dietary Exchanges:
1½ starch

Whole-Grain and Honey Bread

This recipe makes *two* loaves of a basic bread that gets its hearty, chewy texture from bulgur. The bread is great for both sandwiches and toast. If you don't want to bake both loaves at once, you can freeze half of the unbaked dough to use another time.

SERVES 24
1 slice per serving

- ½ cup uncooked bulgur
- ½ cup boiling water
- 2 cups water
- ½ cup honey
- 2 tablespoons canola or corn oil
- 2 teaspoons active dry yeast
- ½ teaspoon salt
- 2 cups bread flour or all-purpose flour
- ¼ cup toasted wheat germ
- 4 cups whole-wheat flour and ½ cup whole-wheat flour, divided use
- Cooking spray

1. In a small bowl, stir together the bulgur and ½ cup boiling water. Let stand for 15 minutes to allow the bulgur to soften.

2. In a large bowl, combine the 2 cups water, honey, oil, yeast, and salt, stirring to dissolve the yeast.

3. Stir in the bread flour, wheat germ, and softened bulgur mixture. Stir in as much of the 4 cups whole-wheat flour as you can until the dough starts to pull away from the side of the bowl.

4. Knead for 6 to 7 minutes, gradually adding, if needed, enough of the remaining ½ cup whole-wheat flour to make the dough smooth and elastic. (The dough shouldn't be dry or stick to the surface. You may not need any of the additional ½ cup whole-wheat flour, or you may need the entire amount if the dough is too sticky.)

5. Using cooking spray, lightly spray a large bowl and a piece of plastic wrap large enough to cover the top of the bowl. Transfer the dough to the bowl, turning to coat all sides with the cooking spray. Cover the bowl with the plastic wrap with the sprayed side down. Let the dough rise in a warm, draft-free place (about 85°F) for 1½ to 2 hours, or until doubled in bulk.

6. Using cooking spray, lightly spray two 8½ x 4½ x 2½-inch loaf pans and 2 pieces of plastic wrap large enough to cover the pans. Punch the dough down. Divide it in half. Shape each half into a loaf. Place each loaf in one of the pans. Cover the pans with the plastic wrap with the sprayed side down. Let the dough rise in a warm, draft-free place for 1½ to 2 hours, or until the dough is 1½ inches higher than the top of the pans.

7. Preheat the oven to 350°F.

8. Bake for 30 minutes, or until the loaves sound hollow when tapped. (Tent the bread with aluminum foil during the last 10 minutes if necessary to prevent overbrowning.) Turn the loaves out onto a cooling rack. Let the bread cool for 15 to 20 minutes before slicing.

9. To freeze one loaf of dough to bake later, follow the preceding directions to the point where you place the shaped dough in a loaf pan. Cover the pan with plastic wrap or aluminum foil, and freeze the dough. After the dough is frozen, about 4 hours, remove it from the pan and wrap it tightly in plastic wrap, then in aluminum foil. When you are ready to bake, unwrap the dough and place it in a sprayed loaf pan. Cover the pan with lightly sprayed plastic wrap with the sprayed side down and let the dough thaw and rise at room temperature in a draft-free place (the thawing and rising will take 4 to 5 hours) or let the dough thaw overnight in the refrigerator and rise as directed. Bake as directed.

PER SERVING

Calories 156
Total Fat 2.0 g
 Saturated Fat 0.0 g
 Trans Fat 0.0 g
 Polyunsaturated Fat 0.5 g
 Monounsaturated Fat 1.0 g
Cholesterol 0 mg
Sodium 51 mg
Carbohydrates 31 g
 Fiber 3 g
 Sugars 6 g
Protein 5 g
Calcium 11 mg
Potassium 114 mg
Dietary Exchanges:
2 starch

Corn Bread Dressing

Too much liquid can make corn bread dressing heavy and gummy, but this recipe has the perfect texture. That's because it calls for adding dried whole-wheat bread and baking the dressing uncovered. Both help the dressing absorb the broth, resulting in a light, flavorful side dish. If you prefer, you can also just enjoy the corn bread on its own.

SERVES 8
½ cup per serving

- Cooking spray
- 4 cups crumbled corn bread (recipe follows)
- 2 slices whole-wheat bread (lowest sodium available), dried and crumbled (about 1½ cups)
- 1 tablespoon olive or canola oil
- ½ cup finely chopped onion
- 1 medium rib of celery, sliced crosswise
- 2 medium garlic cloves, minced
- ¼ cup snipped fresh parsley
- 1½ teaspoons dried summer savory, crumbled
- 1 teaspoon dried thyme, crumbled
- ½ teaspoon pepper
- 1 cup fat-free, low-sodium chicken broth, such as on page 177

1. Preheat the oven to 375°F. Lightly spray a 2-quart glass casserole dish with cooking spray. Set aside.

2. In a large bowl, stir together the corn bread and whole-wheat bread. Set aside.

3. In a large skillet, heat the oil over medium heat, swirling to coat the bottom. Cook the onion, celery, and garlic for 6 to 8 minutes, or until the celery is soft, stirring occasionally.

4. Stir in the remaining ingredients except the broth. Stir into the corn bread mixture. Pour in the broth, stirring until all the dressing is moistened. Transfer to the casserole dish.

5. Bake for 20 to 25 minutes, or until heated through.

PER SERVING
Calories 184
Total Fat 5.5 g
Saturated Fat 0.5 g
Trans Fat 0.0 g
Polyunsaturated Fat 1.0 g
Monounsaturated Fat 3.0 g
Cholesterol 24 mg
Sodium 177 mg
Carbohydrates 29 g
Fiber 2 g
Sugars 3 g
Protein 6 g
Calcium 126 mg
Potassium 169 mg
Dietary Exchanges: 2 starch, ½ fat

Corn Bread

SERVES 12

1 square per serving

Cooking spray

1 cup all-purpose flour

¾ cup yellow or white cornmeal

2 teaspoons baking powder

1 cup fat-free milk

1 large egg

1 tablespoon canola or corn oil

1 tablespoon light tub margarine, melted

1. Preheat the oven to 425°F. Lightly spray an 8-inch square baking pan with cooking spray. Set aside.

2. In a large bowl, stir together the flour, cornmeal, and baking powder.

3. In a small bowl, whisk together the remaining ingredients. Pour all at once into the flour mixture, stirring until the batter is just moistened but no flour is visible. Don't overmix; the batter should be slightly lumpy. Pour into the pan.

4. Bake for 20 to 25 minutes, or until a wooden toothpick inserted in the center comes out clean. Turn out onto a cooling rack. Let cool.

SODIUM SMARTS: Our recipe for corn bread dressing contains about half the sodium of dressing prepared from a packaged mix. Using this homemade corn bread and low-sodium broth helps keep the sodium down.

PER SERVING

Calories 95
Total Fat 2.0 g
Saturated Fat 0.5 g
Trans Fat 0.0 g
Polyunsaturated Fat 0.5 g
Monounsaturated Fat 1.0 g
Cholesterol 16 mg
Sodium 89 mg
Carbohydrates 16 g
Fiber 1 g
Sugars 1 g
Protein 3 g
Calcium 69 mg
Potassium 63 mg
Dietary Exchanges:
1 starch

Zucchini Quick Bread with Nuts and Fruit

Nuts and dried fruit make this attractive bread exceptionally hearty and satisfying, and the zucchini keeps it moist.

SERVES 12
1 slice per serving

- Cooking spray
- 1¼ cups all-purpose flour
- ¼ cup toasted wheat germ
- 1½ teaspoons baking powder
- ½ teaspoon ground cinnamon
- ¼ teaspoon salt
- 1 large egg
- 1 large egg white
- 1 cup shredded zucchini (about 6 ounces)
- ⅔ cup sugar
- ¼ cup canola or corn oil
- 1 teaspoon grated orange zest
- ½ cup chopped walnuts or pecans
- ⅓ cup chopped sweetened dried cranberries or sweetened dried cherries

1. Preheat the oven to 350°F. Lightly spray an 8½ x 4½ x 2½-inch loaf pan with cooking spray. Set aside.

2. In a medium bowl, stir together the flour, wheat germ, baking powder, cinnamon, and salt. Set aside.

3. In a separate medium bowl, using a fork, lightly beat the egg and egg white.

4. Stir the zucchini, sugar, oil, and orange zest into the egg mixture. Add to the flour mixture, stirring just until the batter is moistened but no flour is visible. Don't overmix; the batter should be slightly lumpy. Gently stir in the nuts and cranberries. Spoon into the pan, lightly smoothing the top.

5. Bake for 50 to 55 minutes, or until a wooden toothpick inserted in the center comes out clean. Transfer the bread to a cooling rack. Let stand in the pan for 10 minutes. Turn out onto a cooling rack. Let cool completely, about 2 hours. For maximum flavor, wrap the bread and store overnight at room temperature before slicing.

PER SERVING

Calories 194
Total Fat 8.5 g
Saturated Fat 1.0 g
Trans Fat 0.0 g
Polyunsaturated Fat 4.0 g
Monounsaturated Fat 3.5 g
Cholesterol 16 mg
Sodium 110 mg
Carbohydrates 26 g
Fiber 1 g
Sugars 15 g
Protein 4 g
Calcium 43 mg
Potassium 97 mg
Dietary Exchanges: 2 other carbohydrate, 2 fat

Fried Rice

Instead of buying Chinese take-out fried rice, try making your own. With this flavorful version, you cut the sodium way back, and by using brown rice, you increase the fiber and nutrients.

SERVES 6
½ cup per serving

- 1½ cups uncooked instant brown rice
- 2 large eggs
- 1 teaspoon soy sauce (lowest sodium available) and 2 tablespoons soy sauce (lowest sodium available), divided use
- 1 teaspoon toasted sesame oil
- 1 tablespoon canola or corn oil
- 3 ounces button mushrooms, chopped
- 1 medium garlic clove, minced
- 1 medium carrot, shredded
- ½ cup frozen peas, thawed
- ¼ cup thinly sliced green onions
- 2 tablespoons plain rice vinegar

1. Prepare the rice using the package directions, omitting the salt and margarine. Set aside.

2. Meanwhile, in a small bowl, using a fork, lightly beat the eggs and 1 teaspoon soy sauce.

3. In a small nonstick skillet, heat the sesame oil over medium heat, swirling to coat the bottom. Pour the egg mixture into the hot skillet. Reduce the heat to low. Scramble the eggs until completely set. Coarsely chop the scrambled eggs. Set aside.

4. In a large nonstick skillet, heat the canola oil over medium heat, swirling to coat the bottom. Cook the mushrooms and garlic for 4 to 5 minutes or until soft, stirring occasionally.

5. Stir in the rice, carrot, and peas. Cook for 4 to 6 minutes, or until heated through, stirring occasionally.

6. Stir in the eggs, green onions, rice vinegar, and remaining 2 tablespoons soy sauce. Cook for 1 to 2 minutes, or until heated through.

PER SERVING

Calories 156
Total Fat 5.5 g
Saturated Fat 1.0 g
Trans Fat 0.0 g
Polyunsaturated Fat 1.5 g
Monounsaturated Fat 2.5 g
Cholesterol 62 mg
Sodium 202 mg
Carbohydrates 21 g
Fiber 2 g
Sugars 2 g
Protein 5 g
Calcium 20 mg
Potassium 132 mg
Dietary Exchanges: 1½ starch, 1 fat

MEATS

Processed and cured meats, which include deli meats and packaged sandwich meats, are saturated with sodium. These meats, along with many common meat dishes, such as meat loaf, casseroles, and burgers, are another top source of sodium in Americans' diets. Lean cuts of plain beef are not high in sodium; typical levels range from about 40 mg to about 115 mg for a 3-ounce serving, which is considered a healthy portion. It is how a meat is processed, such as adding marinades or injecting flavorings, that accounts for the level of sodium it contains.

TRY THESE LOWER-SODIUM MEAT RECIPES:

- Smoky Hot Chili con Carne (page 147)
- Beef-and-Broccoli Stir-Fry (page 148)
- Espresso Eye-of-Round (page 150)
- Pork Chops with Sage-Thyme Rub (page 152)

SPOTLIGHT ON: Deli Meats Some of the biggest sodium jolts in meat come from sodium nitrate, a preservative that's used in some processed meats, such as bacon, jerky, and lunch/deli meats. If sandwich meats are in your repertoire, look for lower-sodium varieties or cook your own meats. Limit your use of deli meats to once or twice a week, and keep the amount you stack on your sandwich to no more than 3 ounces. To bulk up your sandwich but add little or no sodium, include baby spinach leaves or dark green lettuce, such as crunchy romaine, and add slices of tomato and cucumber.

SODIUM IN SELECTED MEATS

FOOD	SODIUM (MG)*
bacon, 2 slices	190–370
Canadian bacon, 2 oz	580–800
breakfast sausage, 2 oz	310–400
hot dog, 2 oz	470–635
ham, cured, canned, 2 oz	530
ham, honey-baked, 2 oz	690
ham, deli, 2 oz	690–770
ham, deli, lower-sodium, 2 oz	450–550
salami, 2 oz	480–1,140
roast beef, deli, 2 oz	310–350
Espresso Eye-of-Round (page 150), 3 oz cooked beef	185
ground beef, 95% lean, 4 oz raw (3 oz cooked)	100
cheeseburger, frozen, 3 oz cooked patty	540–580
Smoky Hot Chili con Carne (page 147), 1½ cups	315
flank steak, 4 oz raw (3 oz cooked)	60
beef and broccoli frozen entrée, 9 oz	720–1,660
Beef-and-Broccoli Stir-Fry (page 148), 1 cup beef mixture and ½ cup rice	485
rib roast, 4 oz raw (3 oz cooked)	80
sirloin steak, 4 oz raw (3 oz cooked)	60
pork tenderloin or pork chop, center loin, 4 oz raw (3 oz cooked)	60
Pork Chops with Sage-Thyme Rub (page 152), 3 oz cooked pork	190

***Sodium values have been rounded to the nearest 5 mg.**

SODIUM-SAVING SOLUTIONS

- Processed meats loaded with sodium include luncheon, deli, and cured meats, such as ham, bologna, salami, bacon, Canadian bacon, corned beef, pastrami, liverwurst, hot dogs, sausages, and jerky. They can vary a great deal in sodium content, so be sure to compare nutrition facts panels on the packaging or ask at the deli counter.
- If you do eat processed meats, look for the ones with no nitrates or salt added; if those aren't available, use lower-sodium varieties or consider substituting roast beef and pork you cook at home.
- Marinating meat is a popular technique not only to impart flavor but also to make the meat tender. Bottled marinades, however, usually are full of sodium. (See "Sauces, Gravies, Condiments, and Seasonings.") Instead, try making your own (see recipe on page 214) using table (not cooking) wine, fresh lemon or lime juice, or balsamic vinegar.
- Instead of using bottled marinades, experiment with salt-free dry rubs when grilling, broiling, or baking meats.
- Avoid meat tenderizers; they are high in sodium.
- If using commercial taco kits, toss out the sodium-dense seasoning packets that come with them. Instead, look for a low-sodium variety or flavor the ground beef to taste with garlic powder, onion powder, and chili powder.

Smoky Hot Chili con Carne

The addition of smoked paprika gives this chili a nice, deep flavor that's a little different from that of most other versions.

SERVES 4
1½ cups per serving

Cooking spray

CHILI

- 1 teaspoon canola or corn oil
- 1 pound extra-lean ground beef
- 2 cups water
- 2 cups grape tomatoes
- 1 15.5-ounce can no-salt-added dark red kidney beans or no-salt-added small red beans, rinsed and drained
- 1 cup chopped onion
- 2 medium poblano chiles, seeds and ribs discarded, chopped
- 2 tablespoons chili powder
- 1 tablespoon smoked paprika
- 2 teaspoons ground cumin
- ⅛ to ¼ teaspoon cayenne
- ½ teaspoon salt

⅓ cup snipped fresh cilantro

1. Lightly spray a Dutch oven with cooking spray. Heat the oil over medium-high heat, swirling to coat the bottom. Cook the beef for 3 to 4 minutes, or until browned, stirring occasionally to turn and break it up.

2. Stir in the remaining chili ingredients except the salt. Increase the heat to high and bring to a boil. Reduce the heat and simmer, covered, for 25 minutes, or until the vegetables are tender. Remove from the heat. Stir in the salt.

3. Just before serving, sprinkle the cilantro over the chili.

SODIUM SMARTS: Smoked paprika is a boon to healthy cooking—it provides intense flavor with no salt.

PER SERVING

Calories 314
Total Fat 8.0 g
Saturated Fat 2.5 g
Trans Fat 0.5 g
Polyunsaturated Fat 1.5 g
Monounsaturated Fat 3.0 g
Cholesterol 62 mg
Sodium 316 mg
Carbohydrates 31 g
Fiber 9 g
Sugars 7 g
Protein 34 g
Calcium 108 mg
Potassium 1084 mg
Dietary Exchanges: 1 starch, 3 vegetable, 3 lean meat

Beef-and-Broccoli Stir-Fry

Slightly sweet, slightly nutty, and exploding with color, this classic Asian stir-fry is a feast for both the taste buds and the eyes! This version comes in at only a fraction of the sodium you'd get in many restaurant dishes.

SERVES 4
1 cup beef mixture and ½ cup rice per serving

MARINADE

¼ cup soy sauce (lowest sodium available)

2 tablespoons cider vinegar

1½ tablespoons firmly packed dark brown sugar

1 tablespoon toasted sesame oil

2 teaspoons grated orange zest

¼ teaspoon crushed red pepper flakes

12 ounces flank steak, all visible fat discarded, thinly sliced against the grain, then cut into bite-size pieces

10 ounces frozen brown rice

Cooking spray

1 teaspoon canola or corn oil

2 cups small broccoli florets (about 5 ounces)

CONTINUED

1. In a small glass bowl, whisk together the marinade ingredients. Pour ¼ cup of the marinade into a medium shallow dish. Set aside the marinade remaining in the bowl. Add the beef to the marinade in the dish, turning to coat. Cover and refrigerate for 15 minutes, turning occasionally. Drain the beef, discarding the marinade.

2. Meanwhile, prepare the rice using the package directions. Set aside.

3. Lightly spray a large skillet with cooking spray. Cook the beef over high heat for 2 minutes, or until browned, stirring frequently. Transfer to a medium bowl. Set aside. Wipe the skillet with paper towels, being careful not to burn yourself.

4. Reduce the heat to medium. Pour the oil into the skillet, swirling to coat the bottom. Cook the broccoli, onion, and carrots for 3 minutes, or until the broccoli is tender-crisp, stirring frequently.

5. Stir in the garlic. Cook for 15 seconds.

6. Stir in the beef with any accumulated juices. Increase the heat to medium high and cook for 1 minute, or until the beef is heated through, stirring frequently.

7. Spoon the rice onto plates. Spoon the beef mixture over the rice. Drizzle with the reserved marinade.

- 1 medium onion, cut into 8 wedges
- 1 cup very thinly sliced carrots (about 2 medium, sliced crosswise)
- 2 medium garlic cloves, minced

SODIUM SMARTS: Soy sauce is a very high sodium condiment, coming in at about 1,000 mg per tablespoon. Even though low-sodium soy sauce cuts the sodium by about half, it's still considered a high-sodium product; use it sparingly in your favorite Asian dishes, and avoid adding it at the table.

PER SERVING

Calories 309
Total Fat 10.5 g
Saturated Fat 3.0 g
Trans Fat 0.0 g
Polyunsaturated Fat 1.5 g
Monounsaturated Fat 4.5 g
Cholesterol 40 mg
Sodium 486 mg
Carbohydrates 31 g
Fiber 4 g
Sugars 10 g
Protein 23 g
Calcium 53 mg
Potassium 620 mg
Dietary Exchanges:
1½ starch, 2 vegetable, 3 lean meat

Espresso Eye-of-Round

Instant coffee granules add depth of flavor to this perfectly cooked, perfectly seasoned roast beef—a great solution for avoiding the sodium-laden version available at the deli counter. This flavorful roast provides enough meat for one family dinner and several sandwiches during the week.

SERVES 12
3 ounces beef per serving

- Cooking spray
- 2 teaspoons instant coffee granules (espresso preferred)
- 2 teaspoons dried thyme, crumbled
- 1 teaspoon garlic powder
- 1 teaspoon onion powder
- 1 teaspoon pepper
- 1 teaspoon paprika
- ½ teaspoon salt and ¼ teaspoon salt, divided use
- 1 3-pound eye-of-round roast, all visible fat discarded
- 1 tablespoon olive oil and 1 teaspoon olive oil, divided use

1. Preheat the oven to 325°F. Lightly spray a 13 x 9 x 2-inch pan and its rack with cooking spray (if your pan doesn't have a rack, use a cooling rack). Set aside.

2. In a small bowl, stir together the coffee granules, thyme, garlic powder, onion powder, pepper, paprika, and ½ teaspoon salt.

3. Put the beef on the rack. Rub 1 tablespoon oil all over the beef. Sprinkle the coffee granule mixture all over the beef. Using your fingertips, gently press the mixture so it adheres to the beef.

4. In a large nonstick skillet, heat the remaining 1 teaspoon oil over medium-high heat, swirling to coat the bottom. Cook the beef for 2 minutes on the top and 2 minutes on the bottom, or until browned. Return to the rack.

5. Roast for 1 hour 20 minutes, or until the beef registers 135°F on an instant-read thermometer (don't overcook; the beef won't be done at this point). Transfer the beef to a cutting board. Let stand for 10 minutes to finish cooking (to at least 145°F) and to make slicing easier. Thinly slice the beef. Sprinkle with the remaining ¼ teaspoon salt.

6. Refrigerate leftover beef in an airtight container for up to four days or freeze it for up to one month.

SODIUM SMARTS: Both garlic salt and onion salt are very high in sodium—about 960 mg per teaspoon for the garlic and up to 1,000 mg per teaspoon for the onion. This recipe calls for garlic powder and onion powder, both of which add great flavor but are *sodium free.*

PER SERVING

Calories 144	Carbohydrates 1 g
Total Fat 3.5 g	Fiber 0 g
Saturated Fat 1.0 g	Sugars 0 g
Trans Fat 0.0 g	Protein 25 g
Polyunsaturated Fat 0.5 g	Calcium 258 mg
Monounsaturated Fat 2.0 g	Potassium 9 mg
Cholesterol 48 mg	Dietary Exchanges:
Sodium 186 mg	3 lean meat

Pork Chops with Sage-Thyme Rub

Make it easy on yourself! These pork chops can be seasoned and cooked in about 15 minutes. They're served with a basic au jus that's infused with a powerful medley of herbs and spices from the rub.

SERVES 4
3 ounces pork per serving

- **1 teaspoon garlic powder**
- **1 teaspoon onion powder**
- **½ teaspoon dried sage**
- **½ teaspoon dry mustard**
- **¼ teaspoon dried thyme, crumbled**
- **¼ teaspoon salt**
- **¼ teaspoon pepper**
- **⅛ teaspoon cayenne**
- **4 lean bone-in pork loin chops (about 6 ounces each), all visible fat discarded**
- **1 teaspoon canola or corn oil**
- **½ cup water**

1. In a small bowl, stir together the garlic powder, onion powder, sage, mustard, thyme, salt, pepper, and cayenne. Sprinkle over both sides of the pork. Using your fingertips, gently press the mixture so it adheres to the pork.

2. In a large nonstick skillet, heat the oil over medium-high heat, swirling to coat the bottom. Cook the pork for 4 minutes on each side, or until it registers 145°F on an instant-read thermometer. Remove the skillet from the heat. Let the pork stand in the skillet for 3 minutes. Transfer to plates.

3. Pour the water into the skillet. Bring to a boil over medium-high heat, scraping to dislodge any browned bits. Boil for 1 minute, or until reduced by half, to ¼ cup. Serve over the pork.

SODIUM SMARTS: Season your meats and poultry to perfection with herb rubs, which provide a quick and healthy alternative to the excessive sodium of bottled marinades.

PER SERVING

Calories 161	Carbohydrates 1 g
Total Fat 7.5 g	Fiber 0 g
Saturated Fat 2.0 g	Sugars 0 g
Trans Fat 0.0 g	Protein 20 g
Polyunsaturated Fat 1.0 g	Calcium 28 mg
Monounsaturated Fat 3.5 g	Potassium 284 mg
Cholesterol 51 mg	Dietary Exchanges:
Sodium 191 mg	3 lean meat

POULTRY

Like beef and pork, poultry contains some sodium. Natural, unenhanced poultry contains only 45 to 70 mg of sodium per 3-ounce serving. However, about one-third of the fresh poultry found in grocery store meat cases has been synthetically "enhanced" with a combination of salt, other additives, and water to make the lean poultry meat juicier, tastier, and more tender. Unfortunately, the enhancement adds hundreds of extra milligrams of sodium, so look for unenhanced chicken and add no- or low-sodium seasonings of your choosing. (The recipes in this section use unenhanced, natural chicken and turkey products.)

TRY THESE LOWER-SODIUM POULTRY RECIPES:

- Chicken Parmesan (page 156)
- Country-Fried Chicken (page 157)
- Chicken Pad Thai (page 158)
- Roasted Turkey (page 160)
- Chicken Phyllo Potpie (page 162)
- Crunchy Chicken Nuggets (page 164)

SPOTLIGHT ON: Preseasoned Chicken

How does lemon-herb chicken or garlic-oregano chicken sound for dinner? If chicken (or other poultry or meat) has been seasoned or marinated before being packaged for your convenience, it is loaded with sodium. The more flavor that has been added to a natural food like chicken, the higher your chances of consuming too much sodium. As enticing as these products sound, avoid them to save on sodium. One serving of these flavored specialty chickens can easily have more than 500 mg of sodium, even up to 800 mg—half the daily recommended sodium allowance! Buy your own unenhanced chicken breasts and season them with fresh or dried herbs, garlic, and fresh lemon, and you can re-create the same flavorings with only a fraction of the sodium.

SODIUM IN SELECTED POULTRY

FOOD	SODIUM (MG)*
turkey breast, 4 oz raw (3 oz cooked)	45
turkey breast, deli, 2 oz	470–680
turkey breast, deli, lower-sodium, 2 oz	320
turkey breast, deli, no salt added, 2 oz	30–40
Roasted Turkey (page 160), 3 oz cooked	45
turkey sausage, 2 oz	180–510
chicken breast, 4 oz raw (3 oz cooked)	80
chicken breast, enhanced, 4 oz raw (3 oz cooked)	460
chicken Parmesan, frozen, 11–12 oz	650–1,200
Chicken Parmesan (page 156), 3 oz cooked chicken plus ⅓ cup sauce and ½ cup pasta	365
chicken potpie, frozen, 8 oz	780–1,600
Chicken Phyllo Potpie (page 162), 1 cup chicken mixture	425
chicken nuggets, frozen, 6 pieces, 3 oz	360–590
Crunchy Chicken Nuggets (page 164), 3 oz cooked chicken plus sauce	295
fried chicken with gravy, frozen, 11–13 oz	1,570–1,580
Country-Fried Chicken (page 157), 3 oz cooked chicken plus gravy	420

***Sodium values have been rounded to the nearest 5 mg.**

SODIUM-SAVING SOLUTIONS

- When buying poultry, be sure to check the labels, especially the fine print. Even if the label says "natural"—in any form, such as "100% natural" or "all natural"—the poultry may have been injected with ingredients such as salt, chicken broth, or both. Processors are required to disclose such injections to consumers. The fine print may say something like "contains up to 15% chicken broth"; such wording indicates that the poultry has been enhanced.
- When buying a whole chicken or turkey, avoid those that have been basted or brined. These labels are code for poultry that has had salt added and possibly was injected with preservatives containing sodium. Look for fresh, unprocessed poultry products.
- Pass over any packaged convenience product that has already been seasoned for you. Most of these products, such as marinated chicken breasts or teriyaki-style turkey cutlets, use salt as one of the main ingredients.
- If you eat turkey from the deli or processed turkey often, consider roasting a chicken or turkey and using it for sandwiches.
- If you do eat deli meats, look for the ones with no nitrates or salt added; if those aren't available, use lower-sodium varieties.

Chicken Parmesan

Add extra Mediterranean flair to traditional chicken Parmesan by tossing in grape tomatoes, kalamata olives, and fresh basil at the very end.

SERVES 4
3 ounces chicken, ⅓ cup sauce, and ½ cup pasta per serving

- **4 ounces dried whole-grain spaghetti**
- **4 boneless, skinless chicken breast halves (about 4 ounces each), all visible fat discarded, flattened to ¼-inch thickness**
- **1½ tablespoons fresh lemon juice**
- **¾ cup plain whole-wheat panko**
- **1 teaspoon dried oregano, crumbled**
- **½ teaspoon garlic powder**
- **2 teaspoons olive oil**

SAUCE

- **1 8-ounce can no-salt-added tomato sauce**
- **½ cup grape tomatoes, quartered**
- **8 kalamata olives, chopped**
- **¼ cup chopped fresh basil**

- **¼ cup shredded or grated Parmesan cheese**

1. Prepare the pasta using the package directions, omitting the salt. Drain well in a colander.

2. Meanwhile, brush both sides of the chicken with the lemon juice.

3. In a medium shallow dish, stir together the panko, oregano, and garlic powder. Dip 1 piece of the chicken in the mixture, gently shaking off any excess. Place on a large plate. Using your fingertips, gently press the coating so it adheres to the chicken. Repeat with the remaining chicken.

4. In a large nonstick skillet, heat the oil over medium heat, swirling to coat the bottom. Cook the chicken for 6 minutes on each side, or until lightly browned on the outside and no longer pink in the center.

5. Meanwhile, in a medium saucepan, stir together the tomato sauce and tomatoes. Bring just to a boil over medium-high heat. Reduce the heat and simmer for 2 minutes, or until the tomatoes are soft. Remove from the heat. Stir in the olives and basil. Cover to keep warm. Set aside.

6. Transfer the pasta to plates. Spoon the sauce over the pasta. Place the chicken on top. Sprinkle with the Parmesan.

PER SERVING

Calories 369
Total Fat 9.5 g
Saturated Fat 2.0 g
Trans Fat 0.0 g
Polyunsaturated Fat 1.0 g
Monounsaturated Fat 4.5 g
Cholesterol 76 mg
Sodium 367 mg
Carbohydrates 39 g
Fiber 6 g
Sugars 5 g
Protein 34 g
Calcium 101 mg
Potassium 761 mg
Dietary Exchanges:
2 starch, 1 vegetable, 3 lean meat

Country-Fried Chicken

Serve a little down-home comfort with tender chicken topped with a creamy, peppery gravy that has a hint of thyme.

SERVES 4
3 ounces chicken and 2 tablespoons gravy per serving

- **⅓ cup white whole-wheat flour**
- **1 teaspoon garlic powder**
- **1 teaspoon onion powder**
- **1 teaspoon paprika**
- **1 teaspoon dried thyme, crumbled, and ¼ teaspoon dried thyme, crumbled, divided use**
- **½ teaspoon pepper and ¼ teaspoon pepper, or to taste, divided use**
- **4 boneless, skinless chicken breast halves (about 4 ounces each), all visible fat discarded, flattened to ¼-inch thickness**
- **2 tablespoons canola or corn oil**
- **⅛ teaspoon salt and ¼ teaspoon salt, divided use**
- **2 tablespoons light tub margarine**
- **1 cup fat-free milk**
- **1½ packets (1½ teaspoons) salt-free instant chicken bouillon**

1. In a medium shallow dish, stir together the flour, garlic powder, onion powder, paprika, 1 teaspoon thyme, and ½ teaspoon pepper. Spoon 1 tablespoon of the mixture into a small bowl and set aside.

2. Dip 1 piece of chicken in the remaining flour mixture, turning to coat and gently shaking off any excess. Place on a large plate. Using your fingertips, gently press the mixture so it adheres to the chicken. Repeat with the remaining chicken.

3. In a large nonstick skillet, heat the oil over medium heat, swirling to coat the bottom. Cook the chicken for 6 minutes on each side, or until lightly browned on the outside and no longer pink in the center. Transfer the chicken to a plate, leaving any browned bits in the skillet. Sprinkle the chicken with ⅛ teaspoon salt.

4. Whisk the margarine and reserved 1 tablespoon flour mixture into the skillet. Gradually whisk in the milk, bouillon, remaining ¼ teaspoon thyme, and remaining ¼ teaspoon salt. Bring to a simmer over medium heat. Simmer for 2 minutes, or until thickened, whisking constantly. Spoon the gravy over the chicken. Sprinkle with the remaining ¼ teaspoon pepper.

PER SERVING
Calories 279
Total Fat 12.5 g
Saturated Fat 1.5 g
Trans Fat 0.0 g
Polyunsaturated Fat 3.0 g
Monounsaturated Fat 6.5 g
Cholesterol 74 mg
Sodium 422 mg
Carbohydrates 13 g
Fiber 2 g
Sugars 3 g
Protein 28 g
Calcium 94 mg
Potassium 807 mg
Dietary Exchanges: 1 starch, 3 lean meat, ½ fat

Chicken Pad Thai

Enjoy easy-to-make pad Thai in the comfort of your own home. Our version of the peanutty classic is guaranteed to be a lot healthier, with a lot less sodium, than the restaurant version, and it's just as delicious.

SERVES 4
1½ cups per serving

- 4 ounces whole-grain angel hair pasta or vermicelli, broken in half

SAUCE

- ¼ cup chunky peanut butter (lowest sodium available)
- 3 tablespoons hot water
- 2 tablespoons soy sauce (lowest sodium available)
- 1½ tablespoons fresh lime juice
- 1 tablespoon sugar
- 1 tablespoon plain rice vinegar or white vinegar
- 1 tablespoon minced peeled gingerroot (optional)
- ½ to ¾ teaspoon crushed red pepper flakes
- ¼ teaspoon salt

CONTINUED

1. Prepare the pasta using the package directions, omitting the salt. Drain well in a colander.

2. Meanwhile, in a medium bowl, whisk together the sauce ingredients. Set aside.

3. In a large nonstick skillet, heat the oil over medium-high heat, swirling to coat the bottom. Cook the chicken for 2 to 3 minutes, or until no longer pink in the center, stirring frequently.

4. Stir in the snow peas, carrots, and garlic. Cook for 30 seconds to 1 minute, or until the snow peas are tender-crisp, stirring constantly. Remove from the heat.

5. Stir in the pasta, sauce, green onions, cilantro, and basil. Serve with the lime wedges.

SODIUM SMARTS: Be sure to purchase the plain, not the seasoned, rice vinegar to keep the sodium in check. Plain rice vinegar has about 15 mg of sodium per tablespoon, but seasoned rice vinegar can have between 250 and 550 mg for an equivalent amount. Using seasoned, instead of plain, rice vinegar for this pot of soup could add more than 1,000 mg of unnecessary sodium.

1 teaspoon canola or corn oil

12 ounces boneless, skinless chicken breast halves, all visible fat discarded, cut into thin strips

1 cup fresh or frozen snow peas (about 3 ounces), trimmed if fresh, thawed if frozen, halved diagonally

1 cup matchstick-size carrot strips

4 medium garlic cloves, minced

1 cup finely chopped green onions (about 8 medium)

½ cup snipped fresh cilantro

3 tablespoons chopped fresh basil

1 medium lime, cut into 4 wedges

PER SERVING

Calories 360	Carbohydrates 38 g
Total Fat 12.0 g	Fiber 7 g
Saturated Fat 2.0 g	Sugars 10 g
Trans Fat 0.0 g	Protein 28 g
Polyunsaturated Fat 3.5 g	Calcium 77 mg
Monounsaturated Fat 5.5 g	Potassium 782 mg
Cholesterol 54 mg	Dietary Exchanges:
Sodium 554 mg	2 starch, 2 vegetable, 3 lean meat

Roasted Turkey

Your house will be filled with the inviting aroma of roasting garlic as this turkey cooks. The leftovers make wonderful sandwiches, far superior in flavor to those made from processed deli turkey—and with so much less sodium.

SERVES 14
3 ounces turkey per serving

- Cooking spray
- 2 tablespoons canola or corn oil
- 4 large to extra-large garlic cloves, minced
- 1 teaspoon paprika
- 1 7-pound bone-in turkey breast with skin
- 1 medium orange, cut into 6 wedges
- 1 medium lemon, cut into 6 wedges

1. Preheat the oven to 325°F. Line a roasting pan with aluminum foil. Lightly spray the foil with cooking spray. Set aside.

2. In a small bowl, whisk together the oil, garlic, and paprika.

3. Using your fingers and keeping the skin attached, carefully lift the skin from the meat of the turkey so you can spread 2 tablespoons of the garlic mixture between the skin and the meat. Cover as much area as possible, being careful not to tear the skin. Gently pull the skin back over the top and sides. Using your fingertips, thinly spread the remaining garlic mixture over the outside of the turkey and in the turkey cavity. Place as many of the orange and lemon wedges as possible in the turkey cavity and any remaining fruit in the pan. Place the turkey on the fruit, or if all the fruit fits in the cavity, on the foil.

4. Roast the turkey for 2 to 2½ hours, or until the thickest part of the breast registers 165°F on an instant-read thermometer and the juices run clear. Transfer the turkey to a cutting board. Let stand, lightly covered, for 15 minutes. Discard the skin and any visible fat. If desired, gently squeeze the orange and lemon wedges over the turkey. Discard the wedges. Slice the turkey.

5. Refrigerate leftover turkey in an airtight container for up to four days or freeze in an airtight freezer container for up to two months.

SODIUM SMARTS: When buying poultry, read the labels, especially the fine print, to check whether the product has been "enhanced," "basted," or "brined" with ingredients such as salt or chicken broth, both of which are used to plump it up and increase the flavor. These telltale words clue you in that the poultry has been injected with a salt solution or preservatives containing sodium. Even if poultry is labeled "100% natural" or "all natural," it can contain added sodium in some form, and processors are required to provide this information in a disclosure somewhere on the package.

PER SERVING

Calories 133
Total Fat 2.5 g
Saturated Fat 0.5 g
Trans Fat 0.0 g
Polyunsaturated Fat 0.5 g
Monounsaturated Fat 1.5 g
Cholesterol 71 mg
Sodium 44 mg
Carbohydrates 0 g
Fiber 0 g
Sugars 0 g
Protein 26 g
Calcium 11 mg
Potassium 252 mg
Dietary Exchanges:
3 lean meat

Chicken Phyllo Potpie

Give chicken potpie a light makeover—less sodium and saturated fat and fewer calories—by replacing the usual double piecrust with a top layer of flaky phyllo dough.

SERVES 4
1 cup per serving

- **10 to 12 ounces boneless, skinless chicken breasts, all visible fat discarded**
- **1 tablespoon olive or canola oil**
- **½ cup chopped onion**
- **4 ounces button mushrooms, sliced**
- **3 tablespoons all-purpose flour**
- **1 12-ounce can fat-free evaporated milk**
- **¼ cup fat-free, low-sodium chicken broth, such as on page 177**
- **½ teaspoon dried thyme, crumbled**
- **¼ teaspoon salt**
- **¼ teaspoon pepper**
- **1 cup frozen peas and carrots**
- **4 14 x 9-inch frozen phyllo sheets, thawed**
- **Butter-flavor cooking spray**

1. Preheat the oven to 375°F.

2. Put the chicken in a large nonstick skillet, adding water to cover. Bring to a boil over medium-high heat. Reduce the heat and simmer for 10 to 15 minutes, or until the chicken is no longer pink in the center. Transfer to a cutting board, discarding the liquid.

3. Meanwhile, in a medium saucepan, heat the oil over medium heat, swirling to coat the bottom. Cook the onion for 4 minutes, stirring occasionally. Stir in the mushrooms. Cook for 4 to 5 minutes, or until soft, stirring occasionally.

4. While the chicken and the onion mixture are cooking, put the flour in a medium bowl. Gradually whisk in the evaporated milk. Whisk in the broth, thyme, salt, and pepper. Set aside.

5. When the mushrooms are soft, stir in the flour mixture. Cook for 5 to 6 minutes, or until the sauce is thickened and bubbly, stirring constantly. Set aside.

6. Chop the chicken into bite-size pieces. Stir the chicken and peas and carrots into the sauce. Transfer to an 8- or 9-inch square glass baking dish.

7. Keeping the unused phyllo covered with a damp cloth or damp paper towels to prevent drying, lay a phyllo sheet on a flat surface. Lightly spray the sheet with cooking spray. Working quickly, place a second sheet on top of the first. Lightly spray the second sheet. Continue layering and spraying with the last two sheets. Cut the phyllo stack into 12 smaller stacks. Loosely gather 1 stack and place it on top of the chicken mixture. Repeat with the remaining stacks in a pattern or randomly.

8. Bake for 15 to 20 minutes, or until the filling is bubbly and the phyllo is golden. Let stand for 10 minutes before serving.

SODIUM SMARTS:
Homemade equals healthier when you're avoiding the 780 to 1,600 mg of sodium found in your average frozen single-serve chicken potpie. Our version, with its airy phyllo crust, serves up only 425 mg of sodium per serving.

PER SERVING

Calories 288
Total Fat 6.0 g
  Saturated Fat 1.0 g
  Trans Fat 0.0 g
  Polyunsaturated Fat 1.0 g
  Monounsaturated Fat 3.5 g
Cholesterol 54 mg
Sodium 425 mg
Carbohydrates 31 g
  Fiber 3 g
  Sugars 14 g
Protein 28 g
Calcium 305 mg
Potassium 821 mg
Dietary Exchanges:
1 starch, 1 fat-free milk, 2 lean meat

Crunchy Chicken Nuggets

Panko makes these homestyle chicken nuggets extra crunchy. If you want to turn them into a more kid-friendly dish, omit the cayenne and use the smaller amount of dry mustard in the honey mustard sauce.

SERVES 4
3 ounces chicken and 1 tablespoon sauce per serving

CHICKEN

- **1/3 cup fat-free plain Greek yogurt or low-fat buttermilk**
- **1 medium garlic clove, minced**
- **1 cup plain whole-wheat panko**
- **1 teaspoon dried Italian seasoning, crumbled**
- **1/8 teaspoon cayenne (optional)**
- **1 pound boneless, skinless chicken breasts, all visible fat discarded, cut into 1½-inch cubes**
- **Cooking spray**

SAUCE

- **¼ cup light mayonnaise**
- **2 tablespoons honey**
- **1 to 2 teaspoons dry mustard**
- **½ teaspoon dried parsley, crumbled**
- **¼ teaspoon dried minced onion**

1. Preheat the oven to 450°F.

2. In a shallow dish, stir together the yogurt and garlic. In a separate shallow dish, stir together the panko, Italian seasoning, and cayenne. Set the dishes and a large baking sheet in a row, assembly-line fashion. Dip the chicken in the yogurt mixture, turning to coat. Dip in the panko mixture, turning to coat and gently shaking off any excess. Place the chicken on the baking sheet. Using your fingertips, gently press the mixture so it adheres to the chicken. Lightly spray the top of the chicken with cooking spray.

3. Bake for 15 to 20 minutes, or until the chicken is golden on the outside and no longer pink in the center.

4. Meanwhile, in a small bowl, stir together the sauce ingredients. Drizzle over the cooked nuggets.

PER SERVING
Calories 284
Total Fat 7.5 g
Saturated Fat 1.0 g
Trans Fat 0.0 g
Polyunsaturated Fat 3.0 g
Monounsaturated Fat 1.5 g
Cholesterol 78 mg
Sodium 293 mg
Carbohydrates 25 g
Fiber 2 g
Sugars 10 g
Protein 29 g
Calcium 24 mg
Potassium 513 mg
Dietary Exchanges:
1 starch, ½ other carbohydrate, 3 lean meat

SEAFOOD

Except for shellfish, such as crab, lobster, and shrimp, fish are naturally low in sodium regardless of whether they are the saltwater or the freshwater variety. Choose fish such as salmon, tuna, trout, mackerel, and herring since these are high in omega-3s, which are known to lower cholesterol and blood pressure. Although most shellfish naturally contain higher levels of sodium than most fish, they are good sources of other important vitamins and minerals.

TRY THESE LOWER-SODIUM SEAFOOD RECIPES:

- Parmesan-Garlic Tuna Rotini (page 168)
- Margarita Fish Wraps with Mango Salsa (page 169)
- Shrimp Gumbo (page 170)
- Crunchy Oven-Fried Fish Fillets (page 172)

SPOTLIGHT ON: Canned Tuna Tuna canned in water—what could be healthier than that? After all, tuna is a good source of healthy omega-3 fatty acids, most people in the United States don't eat enough fish, and our bodies need water. One serving—3 ounces—of regular canned tuna can contain about 315 mg of sodium. An equivalent amount of fresh tuna comes in at about 60 mg a serving—about one-fifth of the amount in the canned version—making it clear that the manufacturing process adds the extra sodium. Fortunately, you can now find very low sodium canned tuna, whose sodium equivalent is the same as fresh, for a savings of 270 mg per 3-ounce serving.

SODIUM IN SELECTED SEAFOOD

FOOD	SODIUM (MG)*
salmon, Atlantic, 4 oz raw (3 oz cooked)	60
salmon, canned, 3 oz	345
flounder, 4 oz raw (3 oz cooked)	420
cod, 4 oz raw (3 oz cooked)	80
halibut, 4 oz raw (3 oz cooked)	100
catfish, 4 oz raw (3 oz cooked)	60
trout, 4 oz raw (3 oz cooked)	80
fish fillets, breaded, frozen, 2 oz	250–650
Crunchy Oven-Fried Fish Fillets (page 172), 3 oz cooked fish without sauce	205
tuna, fresh, 4 oz raw (3 oz cooked)	45
tuna, canned, albacore, 3 oz	315
tuna, canned, albacore, lower-sodium, 3 oz	75
tuna, canned, albacore, very low sodium, 3 oz	45
tuna noodle casserole, frozen, 8 oz	515–660
Parmesan-Garlic Tuna Rotini (page 168), 1 cup	355
shrimp, 4 oz raw (3 oz cooked)	225–840
shrimp gumbo, canned, 1 cup	780–795
Shrimp Gumbo (page 170), 1½ cups	395
scallops, 4 oz raw (3 oz cooked)	760
lobster, 4 oz raw (3 oz cooked)	260
crab, 4 oz raw (3 oz cooked)	440

***Sodium values have been rounded to the nearest 5 mg.**

SODIUM-SAVING SOLUTIONS

- When buying canned tuna, choose the very low sodium variety, packed in water.
- Avoid breaded fish fillets, fish sticks, and shellfish because the breadings on these choices are loaded with sodium.
- Because shellfish tend to be higher in sodium than other fish, keep the overall sodium content of the dish down by preparing shellfish with low-sodium ingredients.
- Lemon is a perfect flavor complement for fish, and it's sodium free. When you buy fish, pick up some fresh lemons as well.
- When coating fish to bake or broil, use plain panko mixed with your favorite herbs and no-salt-added seasonings rather than seasoned bread crumbs, which are much higher in sodium.
- Frozen shrimp is often processed with a preservative that greatly increases its sodium content. Some brands can have as much as 840 mg of sodium per serving, so be sure to compare nutrition facts labels to find the lowest-sodium brand available. When you buy "fresh" shrimp at the seafood counter or in a seafood market, find out whether it was frozen (sodium may have been added in the processing) and then thawed.

Parmesan-Garlic Tuna Rotini

A low-sodium twist on traditional tuna casserole, this economical stovetop dish features the heady flavors of Italy—the bite of garlic, the richness of olive oil, and the sharpness of Parmesan cheese.

SERVES 4
1 cup per serving

- 4 ounces dried whole-grain pasta, such as rotini (about 1¼ cups)
- ½ cup frozen green peas
- 1 teaspoon olive oil and 1½ tablespoons olive oil (extra virgin preferred), divided use
- 4 ounces sliced button mushrooms
- 4 medium garlic cloves, minced
- ⅛ to ¼ teaspoon crushed red pepper flakes
- 4 medium green onions, finely chopped
- ½ cup snipped fresh parsley
- ¼ teaspoon salt and ⅛ teaspoon salt, divided use
- 1 4.5-ounce can very low sodium albacore tuna, packed in water, rinsed, well drained, and flaked
- ¼ cup shredded or grated Parmesan cheese

1. Prepare the pasta using the package directions, omitting the salt.

2. Put the peas in a colander. Pour the cooked pasta over the peas. Drain well. Transfer to a large bowl.

3. Meanwhile, in a large nonstick skillet, heat 1 teaspoon oil over medium-high heat, swirling to coat the bottom. Cook the mushrooms for 4 minutes, or until tender, stirring occasionally.

4. Stir in the garlic and red pepper flakes. Cook for 15 seconds. Remove from the heat.

5. Stir the mushroom mixture, green onions, parsley, ¼ teaspoon salt, and remaining 1½ tablespoons oil into the pasta mixture. Sprinkle, in order, with the tuna, remaining ⅛ teaspoon salt, and the Parmesan.

PER SERVING
Calories 244
Total Fat 8.5 g
Saturated Fat 2.0 g
Trans Fat 0.0 g
Polyunsaturated Fat 1.0 g
Monounsaturated Fat 5.0 g
Cholesterol 17 mg
Sodium 354 mg
Carbohydrates 28 g
Fiber 6 g
Sugars 4 g
Protein 17 g
Calcium 98 mg
Potassium 313 mg
Dietary Exchanges:
2 starch, 1½ lean meat, ½ fat

Margarita Fish Wraps with Mango Salsa

Nonalcoholic margarita mix and salt-free jerk seasoning make a tangy, spicy marinade for these fish fillets.

SERVES 4
2 wraps per serving

- 4 thin mild white fish fillets, such as tilapia (about 4 ounces each), rinsed and patted dry
- 1 teaspoon salt-free jerk seasoning blend
- ⅛ teaspoon salt
- ½ cup nonalcoholic liquid margarita mix

SALSA

- 1 15.5-ounce can no-salt-added black beans, rinsed and drained
- 1 large mango, chopped
- 1 medium avocado, chopped
- ¼ cup snipped fresh cilantro
- 2 tablespoons finely chopped fresh jalapeño, seeds and ribs discarded
- 2 tablespoons finely chopped green onions
- 1 tablespoon fresh lime juice
- ½ teaspoon chipotle powder
- ⅛ teaspoon salt

- 8 large butter lettuce leaves

1. Cut the fish lengthwise into strips about ½ inch wide. Arrange in a single layer in a large shallow dish.

2. Sprinkle the seasoning blend and salt over both sides of the fish. Using your fingertips, gently press the seasoning blend so it adheres to the fish. Pour in the margarita mix, turning the fish to coat. Cover and refrigerate for 15 minutes, turning once about halfway through.

3. Meanwhile, in a medium bowl, gently stir together the salsa ingredients. Set aside.

4. When the fish has marinated, drain it and discard the marinade. In a large nonstick skillet, cook the fish over medium-high heat for 1 to 2 minutes on each side, or until it flakes easily when tested with a fork.

5. Fill the lettuce leaves with the fish and salsa. Roll up from the bottom and fold the sides toward the center. Serve immediately.

PER SERVING

Calories 345
Total Fat 9.5 g
Saturated Fat 2.0 g
Trans Fat 0.0 g
Polyunsaturated Fat 1.5 g
Monounsaturated Fat 5.5 g
Cholesterol 57 mg
Sodium 218 mg
Carbohydrates 36 g
Fiber 10 g
Sugars 16 g
Protein 31 g
Calcium 75 mg
Potassium 1209 mg
Dietary Exchanges:
1½ starch, 1 fruit, 3 lean meat

Shrimp Gumbo

Packed with shrimp, veggies, and brown rice, this Louisiana favorite is based on a classic roux (pronounced "roo"). Taking the time to cook the flour and oil together until they are dark brown is worthwhile—the roux will both thicken your gumbo and provide rich flavor.

SERVES 6
1½ cups per serving

- ¼ cup all-purpose flour
- 3 tablespoons canola or corn oil
- ½ cup chopped white onion
- 1 small green or red bell pepper, chopped
- 1 medium rib of celery, sliced
- 2 medium garlic cloves, minced
- 1½ to 2 teaspoons salt-free Cajun seasoning
- ½ teaspoon salt
- 3 cups fat-free, low-sodium chicken broth, such as on page 177
- 8 ounces frozen cut okra (about 1½ cups)
- 1¾ cups water
- 1 cup uncooked instant brown rice
- 1 pound raw medium shrimp in shells, peeled and rinsed
- ⅓ cup snipped fresh parsley

1. In a large saucepan, stir together the flour and oil to make a roux. Cook over medium heat for 12 to 14 minutes, or until a dark reddish brown color (almost as dark as a penny), stirring constantly.

2. Stir in the onion, bell pepper, celery, and garlic. Cook for 8 to 10 minutes, or until tender, stirring frequently.

3. Stir in the Cajun seasoning and salt. Gradually stir in the broth. Stir in the okra. Increase the heat to medium high and bring to a boil. Reduce the heat and simmer for 10 minutes, stirring occasionally.

4. Meanwhile, in a medium saucepan, bring the water to a boil. Stir in the rice. Reduce the heat and simmer, covered, for 10 minutes. Remove the pan from the heat. Set aside, still covered.

5. When the broth mixture is ready, stir in the shrimp. Increase the heat to medium and return to a simmer. Simmer for 4 to 6 minutes, or until the shrimp are pink on the outside, reducing the heat if necessary. Stir in the rice and parsley.

SODIUM SMARTS: To make your own Cajun or Creole seasoning, stir together ½ teaspoon each of chili powder, ground cumin, onion powder, garlic powder, paprika, and pepper, and, if you wish, ⅛ teaspoon of cayenne (this makes just over 1 tablespoon of the blend). Double or triple the amounts and keep the extra blend in a container with a shaker top to use in other dishes.

PER SERVING

Calories 219
Total Fat 8.5 g
Saturated Fat 0.5 g
Trans Fat 0.0 g
Polyunsaturated Fat 2.5 g
Monounsaturated Fat 4.5 g
Cholesterol 95 mg
Sodium 396 mg
Carbohydrates 21 g
Fiber 2 g
Sugars 2 g
Protein 14 g
Calcium 50 mg
Potassium 316 mg
Dietary Exchanges:
1 starch, 1 vegetable, 2 lean meat

Crunchy Oven-Fried Fish Fillets

Crisp on the outside and moist on the inside, these fish fillets "fry" in a small amount of hot oil in the oven. Enjoy them with homemade cocktail sauce that is lower in sodium than its bottled counterpart and is a snap to prepare.

SERVES 4
3 ounces fish and
2 tablespoons cocktail sauce per serving

COCKTAIL SAUCE

- **½ cup no-salt-added ketchup**
- **4 to 6 teaspoons bottled white horseradish, drained**
- **1 teaspoon fresh lemon juice**
- **½ teaspoon Worcestershire sauce (lowest sodium available)**
- **¼ teaspoon salt**

FISH

- **½ cup low-fat buttermilk**
- **2 large egg whites**
- **4 thin mild white fish fillets, such as cod (about 4 ounces each), rinsed and patted dry**
- **½ cup plain panko (lowest sodium available)**
- **2 tablespoons sliced almonds, dry-roasted and finely crushed**

CONTINUED

1. Preheat the oven to 450°F.

2. In a small bowl, stir together the sauce ingredients. Cover and refrigerate for at least 1 hour before serving.

3. In a medium shallow dish, whisk together the buttermilk and egg whites. Add the fish, turning to coat. Cover and refrigerate for 10 minutes to 4 hours (any longer and the texture won't be as good), turning the fish several times if marinating for more than 2 hours. Drain the fish, discarding the buttermilk mixture.

4. Just before baking the fish, in a separate medium shallow dish, stir together the panko, almonds, paprika, dillweed, and pepper.

5. Put the dish with the drained fish, the dish with the panko mixture, and a large plate in a row, assembly-line fashion. Dip 1 piece of fish in the panko mixture, turning to coat and gently shaking off any excess. Place on the plate. Using your fingertips, gently press the coating so it adheres to the fish. Repeat with the remaining fish. Set aside.

6. Pour the oil into an 11 x 7 x 2-inch baking pan, swirling to coat the bottom. Put the pan in the oven for 3 minutes to heat the oil (the oil must be heated before the fish is put in the baking pan or the fish will soak it up too quickly and won't cook properly). Remove from the oven. Arrange the fish in a single layer in the pan.

7. Bake for 4 minutes. Using a flat spatula, carefully turn the fish over. Bake for 2 to 4 minutes, or until the fish flakes easily when tested with a fork. Remove from the oven. Sprinkle the remaining ⅛ teaspoon salt over the fish. For peak flavor and texture, serve immediately with the sauce and lemon wedges.

2 teaspoons paprika
½ teaspoon dried dillweed, crumbled
⅛ teaspoon pepper
2 tablespoons canola or corn oil
⅛ teaspoon salt

---

1 medium lemon, cut into 4 wedges (optional)

SODIUM SMARTS: Panko, or Japanese bread crumbs, is coarser and crunchier than regular bread crumbs, as well as being markedly lower in sodium. Either whole-wheat or plain panko is preferable to seasoned panko to keep your sodium intake down. Plain panko has only about 30 mg of sodium in ¼ cup, compared to an average of 285 mg in the same amount of seasoned panko—although even seasoned panko is preferable to seasoned bread crumbs, which contain, on average, 545 mg of sodium in ¼ cup!

PER SERVING
Calories 254
Total Fat 10.0 g
Saturated Fat 10.0 g
Trans Fat 1.0 g
Polyunsaturated Fat 2.5 g
Monounsaturated Fat 5.5 g
Cholesterol 50 mg
Sodium 380 mg
Carbohydrates 17 g
Fiber 1 g
Sugars 9 g
Protein 25 g
Calcium 77 mg
Potassium 726 mg
Dietary Exchanges:
1 other carbohydrate, 3 lean meat

SOUPS AND BROTHS

Soups can be wonderfully healthy main dishes or side courses, especially when they are chock-full of vegetables and whole grains; however, whether you order soups in a restaurant, purchase the ones that are prepared in the grocery store, or choose the canned variety, these soups can take you off a healthy course when they are also full of sodium. Look at the chart on the next page to compare the huge differences in sodium levels among some common soups and broths.

TRY THESE LOWER-SODIUM SOUP AND BROTH RECIPES:

- Chicken Broth (page 177)
- Beef Broth (page 178)
- Vegetable Broth (page 179)
- Roasted Tomato-Mushroom Bisque with Fresh Basil (page 180)
- Cheddar-Topped Broccoli Soup (page 181)
- Chicken Tortilla Soup with Avocado Pico de Gallo (page 182)
- Hot-and-Sour Soup (page 184)

SPOTLIGHT ON: Broths Chicken, beef, and vegetable broths are kitchen staples in many homes across America and are used as the base for other soups and as flavorful liquid in a wide variety of dishes. Often, however, in commercially prepared versions, much of this flavor comes from salt. By switching to a reduced-sodium, salt-free, or no-salt-added broth, you can save hundreds and hundreds of milligrams of sodium. Especially if you use broths often, consider making them from scratch and freezing them.

SODIUM IN SELECTED SOUPS AND BROTHS

FOOD	SODIUM (MG)*
chicken broth, 1 cup	860–980
chicken broth, 33% less sodium, 1 cup	570
chicken broth, low-sodium, 1 cup	70–140
Chicken Broth (page 177), 1 cup	35
vegetable broth, 1 cup	530–590
Vegetable Broth (page 179), 1 cup	105
beef broth, 1 cup	570–900
beef broth, low-sodium, 1 cup	70–120
Beef Broth (page 178), 1 cup	80
chicken bouillon cube	960–1,150
chicken bouillon, instant, salt-free or very low sodium, 1 tsp	0
beef bouillon cube	610–1,005
beef bouillon, instant, salt-free or very low sodium, 1 tsp	5
broccoli-cheese soup, 1 cup	480
Cheddar-Topped Broccoli Soup (page 181), ⅔ cup (with topping)	175
tomato-basil soup, 1 cup	480–960
Roasted Tomato-Mushroom Bisque with Fresh Basil (page 180), ⅔ cup	150
hot-and-sour soup, 1 cup	875–1,385
Hot-and-Sour Soup (page 184), ½ cup	130
chicken tortilla soup, 1 cup	480–820
Chicken Tortilla Soup with Avocado Pico de Gallo (page 182), 1½ cups	135

***Sodium values have been rounded to the nearest 5 mg.**

SODIUM-SAVING SOLUTIONS

- Many soup manufacturers now make reduced-sodium soups and broths, but because there is a vast difference in the levels of sodium in these products, it is important to compare the nutrition facts panels and choose wisely among the lower-sodium options. In some cases, companies have reduced sodium levels without highlighting the reduction on the front of the package. On the other hand, don't be fooled by soups with names that sound healthy or labels that make them look nutritious.
- When you buy canned soups, take note of the serving sizes. Although some canned soups are intended for one serving each, many others are for two or more servings; if you eat more than the label specifies as a serving, you'll have to multiply the sodium content accordingly.
- When you eat soup in a restaurant, order a cup instead of a bowl; the smaller portion means a smaller amount of sodium.
- If the soup you order in a restaurant arrives with croutons or crackers, eat them sparingly or not at all; both are likely salty additions to the soup, which already is high in sodium.
- Most regular grocery stores carry some reduced-sodium broths, but you can find much lower sodium choices online, in health food stores, or in specialty grocery stores.
- Try making your own broths from scratch and freeze them for future use. If you like to use small amounts of broth for flavoring, you can freeze some of the broth in an ice cube tray. When the cubes are frozen, transfer them to an airtight freezer bag to keep in the freezer. Thaw the cubes in the refrigerator or by heating in the microwave. They'll be readily available anytime you need them. (See our broth recipes on pages 177–179.)
- Avoid most soup mixes and bouillon cubes; they are usually high in sodium.

Chicken Broth

Very flavorful yet very low in sodium, this chicken broth freezes well, making it easy to keep on hand to replace the sodium-laden canned variety. (To freeze broth for later use, see page 176.) You can skip roasting the bones, but the roasting step definitely intensifies the flavor.

MAKES 4 QUARTS
1 cup per serving

- Cooking spray
- 4 pounds chicken bones
- 1 teaspoon canola or corn oil
- 2 medium onions, each quartered
- 2 medium carrots, sliced
- 2 medium leeks (green and white parts), sliced
- 2 medium ribs of celery with leaves, coarsely chopped
- 2 medium garlic cloves
- 2 cups dry white wine (regular or nonalcoholic)
- 5 quarts water
- 6 to 8 sprigs of fresh parsley
- 3 sprigs of fresh thyme or 1 tablespoon dried thyme, crumbled
- 8 whole peppercorns
- 1 or 2 medium dried bay leaves
- 3 whole cloves
- ¼ teaspoon salt

1. Preheat the oven to 400°F. Lightly spray a large baking pan with cooking spray. Put the bones in the pan.

2. Roast for 1 hour, or until browned. (If you prefer a lighter-colored broth, roast for only 30 to 40 minutes.)

3. Meanwhile, in a stockpot, heat the oil over medium-high heat, swirling to coat the bottom. Cook the onions, carrots, leeks, celery, and garlic for 5 minutes, stirring occasionally. Reduce the heat to medium. Cook, covered, for 15 to 20 minutes, or until the leeks are limp.

4. Stir in the wine. Increase the heat to high and bring to a boil. Boil for 5 to 10 minutes, or until the wine has evaporated.

5. Stir in the browned bones and remaining ingredients. Bring to a boil. Reduce the heat and simmer, covered, for 4 to 5 hours. Strain the broth and discard the solids. Cover and refrigerate for at least 8 hours so the flavors blend and the fat rises to the surface. Discard the fat before reheating the broth.

PER SERVING

Calories 13	Carbohydrates 1 g
Total Fat 0.5 g	Fiber 0 g
Saturated Fat 0.0 g	Sugars 0 g
Trans Fat 0.0 g	Protein 2 g
Polyunsaturated Fat 0.0 g	Calcium 5 mg
Monounsaturated Fat 0.0 g	Potassium 100 mg
Cholesterol 0 mg	Dietary Exchanges:
Sodium 37 mg	Free

Beef Broth

Roasting the bones is the key to making this beef broth so flavorful. You'll need to allow plenty of time for this recipe to simmer, but in return you get a heart-healthy, very low sodium broth that can be used in many, many dishes. (To freeze broth for later use, see page 176.)

MAKES 3½ QUARTS
1 cup per serving

- Cooking spray
- 6 pounds beef bones
- 4 medium onions, each cut into 8 wedges
- 4 medium carrots, each cut crosswise into 4 pieces
- 2 medium ribs of celery with leaves, each cut crosswise into 4 pieces
- 6 to 8 medium garlic cloves
- 5 quarts water
- 2½ teaspoons instant coffee granules (optional)
- 6 to 8 sprigs of fresh parsley
- 3 sprigs of fresh thyme or 1 tablespoon dried thyme, crumbled
- 2 medium dried bay leaves
- 8 whole peppercorns
- 3 whole cloves
- ¼ teaspoon salt

1. Preheat the oven to 400°F. Lightly spray a large baking pan with cooking spray.

2. Put the bones, onions, carrots, celery, and garlic in the pan. Lightly spray all with cooking spray.

3. Roast for 40 minutes, or until the bones, vegetables, and garlic are richly browned, turning once halfway through. Transfer to a stockpot. If the bones aren't brown enough, continue roasting them for about 20 minutes.

4. Stir in the remaining ingredients. Bring to a boil over high heat. Reduce the heat and simmer, covered, for 4 to 5 hours. Strain the broth and discard the solids. Cover and refrigerate for at least 8 hours so the flavors blend and the fat rises to the surface. Discard the fat before reheating the broth.

PER SERVING
Calories 10
Total Fat 0.0 g
Saturated Fat 0.0 g
Trans Fat 0.0 g
Polyunsaturated Fat 0.0 g
Monounsaturated Fat 0.0 g
Cholesterol 0 mg
Sodium 82 mg
Carbohydrates 1 g
Fiber 0 g
Sugars 0 g
Protein 2 g
Calcium 10 mg
Potassium 100 mg
Dietary Exchanges: Free

Vegetable Broth

Just a few cloves provide the subtle zing that makes this vegetable broth so good. Try some in other soups and vegetarian dishes or as a substitution for water when cooking rice and other grains. (To freeze broth for later use, see page 176.)

MAKES 3½ QUARTS
1 cup per serving

- 2 teaspoons canola or corn oil
- 2 medium green bell peppers, coarsely chopped
- 4 medium onions, quartered
- 4 large leeks (green and white parts), sliced
- 4½ quarts water
- 4 medium carrots, sliced
- 6 medium ribs of celery with leaves, coarsely chopped
- 2 large tomatoes, halved
- 6 or 7 sprigs of fresh thyme or 2 tablespoons dried thyme, crumbled
- 6 or 7 sprigs of fresh parsley
- 24 whole peppercorns
- 4 medium dried bay leaves
- 6 whole cloves
- ½ teaspoon salt

1. In a stockpot, heat the oil over medium-high heat, swirling to coat the bottom. Cook the bell pepper for 3 minutes, stirring occasionally. Stir in the onions and leeks. Cook for 4 to 5 minutes, or until the edges of the bell pepper are richly browned, stirring occasionally.

2. Stir in the remaining ingredients. Increase the heat to high and bring to a boil. Reduce the heat and simmer for 1 hour 15 minutes to 1 hour 30 minutes. Strain the broth and discard the solids. Cover and refrigerate for at least 8 hours so the flavors blend.

PER SERVING
Calories 11
Total Fat 0.5 g
Saturated Fat 0.0 g
Trans Fat 0.0 g
Polyunsaturated Fat 0.0 g
Monounsaturated Fat 0.5 g
Cholesterol 0 mg
Sodium 103 mg
Carbohydrates 1 g
Fiber 0 g
Sugars 0 g
Protein 0 g
Calcium 3 mg
Potassium 23 mg
Dietary Exchanges: Free

Roasted Tomato-Mushroom Bisque with Fresh Basil

Roasted vegetables are the key to this thick and creamy soup's delicious depth of flavor, which is why so little salt is needed.

SERVES 6
⅔ cup per serving

- 2 pounds tomatoes (about 6 medium), seeded and coarsely chopped
- 8 ounces button mushrooms, sliced
- ½ cup chopped onion
- 2 large garlic cloves
- 2 tablespoons olive oil
- ¼ teaspoon salt
- ¼ teaspoon pepper
- 1½ cups fat-free, low-sodium chicken or vegetable broth, such as on pages 177 and 179
- 1 5-ounce can fat-free evaporated milk
- ¼ cup snipped fresh basil and (optional) 2 teaspoons snipped fresh basil, divided use
- ¼ cup fat-free plain Greek yogurt

1. Preheat the oven to 450°F.

2. Place the tomatoes, mushrooms, onion, and garlic in a baking pan large enough to hold them in a single layer. Drizzle with the oil. Toss to coat. Sprinkle with the salt and pepper.

3. Roast for 40 to 45 minutes, or until lightly browned, stirring once halfway through.

4. In a food processor or blender (vent the blender lid), process the tomato mixture and broth until smooth. Pour into a large saucepan.

5. Stir in the evaporated milk and ¼ cup basil. Cook over medium heat for 5 to 10 minutes, or until heated through. To serve, spoon a dollop of yogurt onto each serving. Sprinkle the remaining 2 teaspoons basil, if using, on the yogurt.

PER SERVING

Calories 110
Total Fat 5.0 g
  Saturated Fat 0.5 g
  Trans Fat 0.0 g
  Polyunsaturated Fat 0.5 g
  Monounsaturated Fat 3.5 g
Cholesterol 1 mg
Sodium 150 mg
Carbohydrates 12 g
  Fiber 3 g
  Sugars 9 g
Protein 6 g
Calcium 109 mg
Potassium 639 mg
Dietary Exchanges:
2 vegetable, ½ fat-free milk, 1 fat

Cheddar-Topped Broccoli Soup

This soup still gives you the rich flavor and creaminess you expect from broccoli-cheese soup, but you'll save big on sodium, calories, and saturated fat compared to what you'd have with restaurant or canned versions.

SERVES 6
⅔ cup soup plus scant 1 tablespoon topping per serving

SOUP

- 1 teaspoon olive oil and 2 teaspoons olive oil (extra virgin preferred), divided use
- 1 cup diced onion
- 2 medium garlic cloves, minced
- 2½ cups fat-free, low-sodium vegetable broth, such as on page 179
- 14 ounces frozen broccoli florets
- ½ teaspoon dried thyme, crumbled
- ½ teaspoon dry mustard
- ⅛ teaspoon cayenne
- 2 tablespoons light tub cream cheese

TOPPING

- ¼ cup snipped fresh parsley
- ¼ cup shredded low-fat sharp Cheddar cheese
- ⅛ teaspoon salt
- ⅛ teaspoon pepper

1. In a large saucepan, heat 1 teaspoon oil over medium heat, swirling to coat the bottom. Cook the onion for 5 minutes, or until golden, stirring frequently.

2. Stir in the garlic. Cook for 15 seconds.

3. Stir in the broth, broccoli, thyme, mustard, and cayenne. Increase the heat to high and bring to a boil. Reduce the heat and simmer, covered, for 8 to 10 minutes, or until the broccoli is tender.

4. In a food processor or blender (vent the blender lid), process the soup in batches until smooth. Return the soup to the pan.

5. Stir in the cream cheese and remaining 2 teaspoons oil. Cook over medium heat for 1 minute, or until the cream cheese has melted, stirring constantly. Remove from the heat.

6. In a small bowl, lightly toss together the topping ingredients. Sprinkle over the soup.

PER SERVING
Calories 76
Total Fat 4.0 g
Saturated Fat 1.0 g
Trans Fat 0.0 g
Polyunsaturated Fat 0.5 g
Monounsaturated Fat 2.0 g
Cholesterol 4 mg
Sodium 175 mg
Carbohydrates 7 g
Fiber 3 g
Sugars 2 g
Protein 4 g
Calcium 88 mg
Potassium 223 mg
Dietary Exchanges:
1 vegetable, 1 fat

Chicken Tortilla Soup with Avocado Pico de Gallo

Even dishes as popular as tortilla soup can sometimes benefit from a bit of change, especially when that change helps to reduce the sodium. In this version, black beans are added to the soup and a version of fresh pico de gallo with avocado is sprinkled on top. The soup is so flavorful that you won't need to add any salt at all.

SERVES 6
1½ cups per serving

SOUP

- **1 pound boneless, skinless chicken breasts, all visible fat discarded**
- **1 tablespoon canola or corn oil**
- **½ cup chopped onion**
- **2 medium garlic cloves, minced**
- **1 14.5-ounce can no-salt-added diced tomatoes, undrained**
- **3 6-inch corn tortillas, coarsely chopped or torn**
- **2 tablespoons no-salt-added tomato paste**
- **2 tablespoons finely chopped fresh jalapeño, seeds and ribs discarded**
- **3 cups fat-free, low-sodium chicken broth, such as on page 177**
- **1 15.5-ounce can no-salt-added black beans, rinsed and drained**

CONTINUED

1. Put the chicken in a large nonstick skillet, adding water to cover. Bring to a boil over medium-high heat. Reduce the heat and simmer for 10 to 15 minutes, or until the chicken is no longer pink in the center. Transfer to a cutting board, discarding the liquid. Set aside.

2. In a large saucepan, heat the oil over medium heat, swirling to coat the bottom. Cook the onion and garlic for 4 minutes, or until soft, stirring occasionally.

3. Stir in the tomatoes with liquid, tortillas, tomato paste, and jalapeño. Cook for 5 minutes, stirring constantly. Pour into a food processor or blender (vent the blender lid) and process until smooth. Return to the pan.

4. Chop the chicken. Stir the chicken, broth, and beans into the tomato mixture. Bring to a boil over high heat. Reduce the heat and simmer for 15 minutes.

5. Meanwhile, in a medium bowl, stir together the pico de gallo ingredients. Serve sprinkled over the soup.

SODIUM SMARTS: Most canned tomato products contain a great deal of sodium, but using no-salt-added tomato products will save you hundreds of milligrams of sodium. For instance, this recipe calls for one 14.5-ounce can of no-salt-added tomatoes, which contains about 55 mg of sodium. If you used the same size can of regular tomatoes instead, you could increase the sodium content by as much as 800 mg or more, or 15 times as much!

PICO DE GALLO

- 1 small avocado, chopped
- 1 medium tomato, seeded and finely chopped
- ¼ cup thinly sliced green onions
- 2 tablespoons snipped fresh cilantro
- 1 tablespoon fresh lime juice

PER SERVING

Calories 272
Total Fat 8.0 g
Saturated Fat 1.0 g
Trans Fat 0.0 g
Polyunsaturated Fat 1.5 g
Monounsaturated Fat 5.0 g
Cholesterol 48 mg
Sodium 136 mg
Carbohydrates 26 g
Fiber 7 g
Sugars 8 g
Protein 23 g
Calcium 71 mg
Potassium 1031 mg
Dietary Exchanges: 1 starch, 2 vegetable, 2½ lean meat

Hot-and-Sour Soup

This soup gets its "hot" from the chili paste and its "sour" from the rice vinegar.

SERVES 8
½ cup per serving

- **1½ teaspoons canola or corn oil**
- **2 ounces shiitake mushrooms, stems discarded, sliced**
- **1½ teaspoons grated peeled gingerroot**
- **1 medium garlic clove, minced**
- **½ to 1 teaspoon red chili paste or hot chili sauce**
- **3 cups fat-free, low-sodium chicken or vegetable broth, such as on pages 177 and 179**
- **½ 8-ounce can bamboo shoots, drained and coarsely chopped**
- **2 tablespoons soy sauce (lowest sodium available)**
- **2 tablespoons plain rice vinegar**
- **¼ teaspoon sugar**
- **1 tablespoon cornstarch**
- **2 tablespoons water**
- **1 small egg, lightly beaten with a fork**
- **¼ cup snipped fresh cilantro**
- **2 tablespoons chopped green onions**

1. In a medium saucepan, heat the oil over medium heat, swirling to coat the bottom. Cook the mushrooms, gingerroot, garlic, and chili paste for 4 to 5 minutes, or until the mushrooms are soft, stirring occasionally.

2. Stir in the broth, bamboo shoots, soy sauce, vinegar, and sugar. Increase the heat to high and bring to a boil. Reduce the heat and simmer for 10 minutes.

3. Put the cornstarch in a small bowl. Add the water, whisking to dissolve. Stir into the soup.

4. Stir the soup in one direction so it swirls, and slowly pour in the egg in a steady stream. The egg will cook almost immediately and form ribbons. Pour into bowls. Serve sprinkled with the cilantro and green onions.

PER SERVING

Calories 30
Total Fat 1.5 g
Saturated Fat 0.0 g
Trans Fat 0.0 g
Polyunsaturated Fat 0.5 g
Monounsaturated Fat 0.5 g
Cholesterol 18 mg
Sodium 129 mg
Carbohydrates 3 g
Fiber 0 g
Sugars 1 g
Protein 2 g
Calcium 8 mg
Potassium 94 mg
Dietary Exchanges:
½ fat

CHEESE AND OTHER DAIRY PRODUCTS

Cheese is a much-loved and nutritious food, yet because of its universal popularity, it also can add a huge amount of sodium to the average American diet. All cheeses contain some salt, which is needed to produce as well as preserve the cheese; some cheeses, such as feta, blue, and American, have much higher sodium contents than others, such as Swiss, Cheddar, and Colby. With the exception of buttermilk and cheese, most dairy products do not contain added salt, although most contain some naturally occurring sodium, and some contain sodium additives. When buying dairy products, be sure to read labels and choose the lower-sodium products.

TRY THESE LOWER-SODIUM CHEESE-BASED RECIPES:

- Family Night Lasagna (page 188)
- Cheddar-Topped Beef-and-Veggie Enchiladas (page 190)
- Veggie Mac and Cheese (page 192)

SPOTLIGHT ON: Low-Fat Cottage Cheese

Although low-fat cottage cheese is a great source of calcium and protein, it also provides a large amount of sodium. A half-cup serving of 1 or 2 percent low-fat cottage cheese can contain about 460 mg of sodium—nearly one-third of the American Heart Association's recommended amount of sodium for an entire day.

SODIUM IN SELECTED CHEESE AND OTHER DAIRY PRODUCTS

FOOD	SODIUM (MG)*
mozzarella cheese, whole-milk, 1 oz	120
mozzarella cheese, part-skim, 1 oz	175
Parmesan cheese, 1 oz	435
ricotta cheese, whole-milk, 1 oz	25
Cheddar cheese, 1 oz	175
Cheddar cheese, low-fat, 1 oz	175
Cheddar cheese, fat-free, 1 oz	220–285
American cheese, 1 oz	355–470
American cheese, low-fat, 1 oz	385–475
American cheese, fat-free, 1 oz	435
Swiss cheese, 1 oz	55
Swiss cheese, low-fat, 1 oz	75
feta cheese, 1 oz	315
feta cheese, low-fat, 1 oz	370–390
blue cheese, 1 oz	395
Colby cheese, 1 oz	180
cream cheese, 1 oz	90
cottage cheese, 1 oz	105
cottage cheese, low-fat, 1 oz	115
cottage cheese, fat-free, 1 oz	95
sour cream, 2 tbsp	10–45
sour cream, light, 2 tbsp	20
sour cream, fat-free, 2 tbsp	25–50
margarine, 1 tsp	35
buttermilk, low-fat, 8 oz	255
half-and-half, 2 tbsp	10
half-and-half, fat-free, 2 tbsp	25–45
milk, fat-free, 8 oz	105

FOOD	SODIUM (MG)*
milk, 2%, 8 oz	115
milk, whole, 8 oz	105
yogurt, plain, whole-milk, 8 oz	115
yogurt, plain, fat-free, 8 oz	150–190
yogurt, Greek, plain, fat-free, 8 oz	85
ice cream, vanilla, fat-free, ½ cup	45–70
macaroni and cheese, mix, 1 oz	215–270
Veggie Mac and Cheese (page 192), ½ cup	160

***Sodium values have been rounded to the nearest 5 mg.**

SODIUM-SAVING SOLUTIONS

- Natural cheeses are salty, but choose them over cheese products and processed cheeses, which are even saltier.
- Because cottage cheese is very high in sodium, consider substituting fat-free Greek yogurt for a snack or breakfast and substituting ricotta cheese in recipes.
- Be aware that although lower-fat dairy products are lower in calories and saturated fat, they tend to be higher in sodium than their higher-fat counterparts.
- Sodium-heavy cheeses, such as Parmesan or Romano, are often companions to pasta, so be mindful of how much you use. Think of cheese more as a garnish than as a topping so that you will use a light dusting of it rather than a downpour.

Family Night Lasagna

This fresh take on a cheesy classic pares down the sodium and saturated fat for a comfort food that is both satisfying and heart healthy.

SERVES 8
one 3 x 4½-inch piece per serving

Cooking spray
8 ounces whole-grain lasagna noodles
1 pound extra-lean ground beef
8 ounces button mushrooms, sliced
1 cup chopped onion
3 medium garlic cloves, minced
3 cups no-salt-added tomato sauce
2 tablespoons dried Italian seasoning
¼ teaspoon crushed red pepper flakes
2 cups fat-free ricotta cheese
1 cup shredded or grated Parmesan cheese
2 cups shredded low-fat mozzarella cheese

1. Preheat the oven to 375°F. Lightly spray a 13 x 9 x 2-inch glass baking dish with cooking spray.

2. Prepare the noodles using the package directions, omitting the salt.

3. Meanwhile, in a large nonstick skillet, stir together the beef, mushrooms, onion, and garlic. Cook over medium-high heat for 8 to 10 minutes, or until the beef is browned on the outside and no longer pink in the center, stirring occasionally to turn and break up the beef. Reduce the heat to low. Cook, covered, for 3 to 4 minutes, or until the mushrooms have released their liquid. Increase the heat to high. Cook, uncovered, for 2 to 3 minutes, or until the liquid has evaporated.

4. Stir in the tomato sauce, Italian seasoning, and red pepper flakes. Reduce the heat to low. Cook for 5 to 6 minutes, or until heated through.

5. In a large bowl, stir together the ricotta and Parmesan.

6. In the baking dish, layer one-third of the cooked noodles, half of the ricotta mixture, one-third of the beef mixture, and one-third of the mozzarella. Repeat the layers. Finish in order with the remaining noodles, beef mixture, and mozzarella.

7. Bake, covered, for 35 to 40 minutes, or until the lasagna is heated through and the mozzarella is melted.

SODIUM SMARTS: Just by substituting no-salt-added tomato sauce for the regular kind in this recipe, you save hundreds of milligrams of sodium per serving.

PER SERVING

Calories 377
Total Fat 9.0 g
Saturated Fat 4.0 g
Trans Fat 0.0 g
Polyunsaturated Fat 0.5 g
Monounsaturated Fat 3.5 g
Cholesterol 58 mg
Sodium 491 mg
Carbohydrates 38 g
Fiber 6 g
Sugars 10 g
Protein 34 g
Calcium 499 mg
Potassium 707 mg
Dietary Exchanges:
2 starch, 2 vegetable, 4 lean meat

Cheddar-Topped Beef-and-Veggie Enchiladas

Although the list of ingredients for these enchiladas is fairly long, the preparation isn't complicated. This one-dish meal is much lower in sodium, saturated fat, and calories than a similar dish from a Tex-Mex restaurant.

SERVES 4
2 enchiladas per serving

Cooking spray

SAUCE

1 8-ounce can no-salt-added tomato sauce
2 tablespoons water
2 teaspoons ground cumin
2 teaspoons cider vinegar
1 teaspoon sugar
¼ teaspoon salt
⅛ teaspoon cayenne

FILLING

12 ounces extra-lean ground beef
1 cup chopped onion
1 large green bell pepper, chopped
1 medium yellow summer squash, chopped
1 tablespoon chili powder
2 teaspoons ground cumin
⅛ teaspoon salt

CONTINUED

1. Preheat the oven to 350°F. Lightly spray a 13 x 9 x 2-inch glass baking dish and a large skillet with cooking spray. Set aside.

2. In a small bowl, stir together the sauce ingredients. Set aside.

3. In the large skillet, cook the beef over medium-high heat for 2 minutes, stirring occasionally to turn and break up the beef.

4. Stir in the onion, bell pepper, and summer squash. Cook for 3 minutes, or until the onion is soft, stirring frequently. Stir in the chili powder, remaining 2 teaspoons cumin, and ⅛ teaspoon salt.

5. Lightly brush one-third of the sauce on both sides of the tortillas, placing them on a large flat surface, such as a long piece of wax paper on the counter, as you finish. Spoon the filling down the center of each tortilla, leaving a half-inch border at the top and the bottom. Roll up jelly-roll style. Place with the seam down in the baking dish.

6. Bake, covered, for 25 minutes. Spoon the remaining two-thirds of the sauce over the enchiladas. Sprinkle, in order, with the final ⅛ teaspoon salt, the cilantro, and the Cheddar. Bake, uncovered, for 5 minutes, or until the Cheddar melts.

8 6-inch corn tortillas
⅛ teaspoon salt
⅓ cup snipped fresh cilantro
¾ cup shredded low-fat sharp Cheddar cheese

SODIUM SMARTS: Bypassing flour tortillas and using corn tortillas instead can shave off about 140 mg of sodium per tortilla.

PER SERVING

Calories 284
Total Fat 7.5 g
  Saturated Fat 3.0 g
  Trans Fat 0.5 g
  Polyunsaturated Fat 1.0 g
  Monounsaturated Fat 2.5 g
Cholesterol 51 mg
Sodium 577 mg
Carbohydrates 28 g
  Fiber 5 g
  Sugars 8 g
Protein 27 g
Calcium 195 mg
Potassium 782 mg
Dietary Exchanges:
1 starch, 3 vegetable, 3 lean meat

Veggie Mac and Cheese

Try this lower-sodium version of the family favorite—it's almost as easy as the boxed variety but has less sodium plus extra nutrients and color. Adding the saltier ingredients at the end of cooking retains their flavor, allowing you to use less and taste them more.

SERVES 4
½ cup per serving

- ½ cup dried whole-grain elbow macaroni or penne (about 2 ounces)
- ¾ cup small broccoli florets
- ½ medium red bell pepper, chopped
- ⅔ cup fat-free milk
- 1 tablespoon all-purpose flour
- ¼ teaspoon Worcestershire sauce (lowest sodium available)
- Dash of cayenne, or to taste
- ¼ cup shredded low-fat sharp Cheddar cheese
- 1 tablespoon shredded or grated Parmesan cheese
- ⅛ teaspoon salt

1. Prepare the pasta using the package directions, omitting the salt and stirring in the broccoli and bell pepper during the last 3 minutes of cooking. Drain well in a colander.

2. About 10 minutes after putting the water on to boil for the pasta, in a medium saucepan, whisk together the milk, flour, Worcestershire sauce, and cayenne. Cook over medium heat for 1 to 2 minutes, or until thickened, whisking constantly. Remove from the heat.

3. Stir the pasta mixture into the sauce. Sprinkle with the Cheddar, stirring to combine. Transfer to a serving bowl. Sprinkle with the Parmesan and salt. Don't stir.

PER SERVING
Calories 100
Total Fat 1.5 g
Saturated Fat 0.5 g
Trans Fat 0.0 g
Polyunsaturated Fat 0.0 g
Monounsaturated Fat 0.5 g
Cholesterol 3 mg
Sodium 161 mg
Carbohydrates 16 g
Fiber 2 g
Sugars 4 g
Protein 6 g
Calcium 181 mg
Potassium 107 mg
Dietary Exchanges:
1 starch, ½ lean meat

SNACKS

Do you ever think of a snack as "just a little something" to hold you over until the next meal? The problem is that, depending on what you choose, snacking on several small amounts can add a lot to your daily sodium intake, especially if you grab two or three snacks throughout the day. Even what you think are healthy snacks, such as nuts or granola bars, can be salt traps. It may not come as much of a surprise that many snack items are salty, but do you really know how much sodium lurks in *your* snacks? Check out the chart on the next page to see.

TRY THESE LOWER-SODIUM SNACK RECIPES:

- Hot Soft Pretzels (page 196)
- Three-Way Popcorn (page 198)
- Granola Mini Bars (page 200)
- Italian-Style Tortilla Chips (page 201)
- Herbed Veggie Chips (page 202)
- White Bean, Kalamata, and Basil Hummus (page 204)
- Nutty Cereal-and-Seeds Snack Mix (page 205)

SPOTLIGHT ON: Pretzels In general, the individual snack-size bags you find in the vending machine weigh 1 to 2 ounces. That may not seem like much food, but those snacks may be loaded with sodium. Pretzels, one of the most traditional snack foods, are among the worst offenders. A 1-ounce serving of pretzels can contain about 500 mg of sodium—one-third of the daily recommended amount.

SODIUM IN SELECTED SNACKS

FOOD	SODIUM (MG)*
potato chips, regular, 1 oz	150–190
potato chips, baked, 1 oz	150–200
potato chips, barbecue, 1 oz	190–215
Herbed Veggie Chips (page 202), 1 oz	55
tortilla chips, 1 oz	80–150
Italian-Style Tortilla Chips (page 201), 8 chips	25
pretzels, salted, 1 oz	385–620
pretzels, unsalted, 1 oz	80–100
Hot Soft Pretzels (page 196), 1 pretzel	60
hummus, ¼ cup	235–400
White Bean, Kalamata, and Basil Hummus (page 204), ¼ cup	130
cheese puffs, 1 oz	255–370
beef jerky, 1 oz	585–600
pork skins, 1 oz	515–630
peanuts, salted, 1 oz	90–230
peanuts, unsalted, 1 oz	0
pumpkin seeds, salted, 1 oz	75
pumpkin seeds, unsalted, 1 oz	0–5
snack mix, ½ cup	210–330
Nutty Cereal-and-Seeds Snack Mix (page 205), ⅓ cup	70
granola/cereal bar, 1 oz	65–120
Granola Mini Bars (page 200), 1 2-inch square	85
popcorn, microwave, light, 1 oz	220–420
Three-Way Popcorn with Lemon-Herb Seasoning (page 198), 2 cups	0
crackers, 1 oz	180–315

***Sodium values have been rounded to the nearest 5 mg.**

SODIUM-SAVING SOLUTIONS

- When you buy individually packaged snack items, be aware of the serving sizes. You might logically assume that these snack-size bags hold one serving each, but some actually hold two or more servings. If this is the case with your snack and you are going to eat all the contents, you need to multiply the sodium amount on the nutrition facts panel by the number of servings to know how much sodium you are actually consuming.
- When buying pretzels, choose unsalted varieties. If you want to give them a flavor boost, coat them very lightly with low-sodium peanut butter, another low-sodium nut butter, or low-sodium mustard.
- When shopping for crackers, buy reduced-sodium whole-grain varieties. Be sure to compare nutrition facts panels and choose crackers with the best possible combination of low sodium and high fiber content. Also, check the ingredient list to see whether a whole grain is listed first; that information, not the marketing hype on the front of the package, will tell you whether the crackers are indeed whole grain.
- Incorporate fat-free yogurt and fresh or dried fruit into your snack repertoire to replace commercially packaged snack products.
- When you're hungry for snack food, you may be craving texture or crunch more than just saltiness. Instead of reaching for the chips or pretzels, try a small handful (about 1½ ounces) of unsalted nuts. For more intense flavor, try dry-roasting unsalted nuts, such as pecans, almonds, or walnuts, either in a skillet or in the oven. Take them off the heat as soon as you smell the nutty aroma and lightly spray them with cooking spray. You can sprinkle them with cayenne or chili powder for a spicy kick or cinnamon or pumpkin pie spice for a sweeter flavor. Make extra to add to salads and oatmeal.
- If you sit in front of the TV with a big bag of chips or pretzels, you most likely will eat more than one serving, which can up your sodium intake considerably. Instead, keep temptation at bay and your sodium intake in check by dividing large bags of snacks into single servings and putting those in individual airtight plastic bags.

Hot Soft Pretzels

Most pretzels are high in sodium because salt is not only on the outside but in the dough as well. With this recipe for one dough and two topping options, you can easily please all soft-pretzel lovers. Choose sesame, poppy, and caraway seeds for savory pretzels; if you're more in the mood for something sweet, go with the cinnamon-sugar topping.

SERVES 12
1 pretzel per serving

PRETZELS

- **1 cup lukewarm fat-free milk (105°F to 115°F)**
- **2 teaspoons active dry yeast**
- **2 tablespoons sugar**
- **2 tablespoons olive oil**
- **¼ teaspoon salt**
- **1½ cups whole-wheat flour**
- **1 cup bread flour, 3 to 4 tablespoons bread flour, and ½ cup bread flour, divided use**
- **Cooking spray**
- **1 large egg yolk**
- **2 tablespoons water**

THREE-SEED TOPPING

- **1 tablespoon sesame seeds**
- **1 tablespoon poppy seeds**
- **1 teaspoon caraway seeds, crushed**

CINNAMON-SUGAR TOPPING

- **¼ cup sugar**
- **½ teaspoon ground cinnamon**

1. In a medium bowl, combine the milk and yeast, stirring to dissolve. Let stand for 5 minutes.

2. Stir in the 2 tablespoons sugar, the oil, and the salt. Add the whole-wheat flour and 1 cup bread flour, stirring until the dough starts to pull away from the side of the bowl.

3. Using the 3 to 4 tablespoons of bread flour, lightly flour a flat surface. Turn out the dough. Knead for 6 to 7 minutes, gradually adding, if needed, enough of the remaining ½ cup bread flour to make the dough smooth and elastic. (The dough shouldn't be dry or stick to the surface. You may not need any of the additional ½ cup bread flour, or you may need the entire amount if the dough is too sticky.)

4. Using cooking spray, lightly spray a large bowl and a piece of plastic wrap large enough to cover the top of the bowl. Transfer the dough to the bowl, turning to coat all sides with the cooking spray. Cover the bowl with the plastic wrap with the sprayed side down. Let the dough rise in a warm, draft-free place (about 85°F) for about 1 hour, or until doubled in bulk.

5. Preheat the oven to 400°F. Line a large baking sheet with cooking parchment. Set aside.

6. Punch the dough down. Divide it into 12 equal pieces. Using a small amount of bread flour, lightly flour a flat surface. Roll each piece of dough into an 18-inch rope. Working with one rope, at a point about 4 inches from each end, cross one end of the rope over the other to form a circle with two 4-inch-long tails. Bring the tails together and twist them once. Lift the twist, folding the dough to the opposite side of the circle so that the tails slightly overlap the circle, giving it the shape of a pretzel. Place the pretzel on the baking sheet. Repeat with the remaining dough ropes, spacing the pretzels 1 inch apart. Set aside.

7. In a small bowl, using a fork, beat the egg yolk and water together. Set aside.

8. In a separate small bowl, stir together the ingredients for either topping.

9. Brush the yolk mixture over the top of the pretzels. Sprinkle the pretzels with the topping.

10. Bake for 15 minutes, or until golden brown. Serve hot. Transfer leftovers to a cooling rack. Let cool completely, about 1 hour.

11. Store in an airtight container for up to three days. To reheat, microwave on 100 percent power (high) for 20 seconds.

PER SERVING

THREE-SEED TOPPING

Calories 143
Total Fat 4.0 g
Saturated Fat 0.5 g
Trans Fat 0.0 g
Polyunsaturated Fat 1.0 g
Monounsaturated Fat 2.0 g
Cholesterol 16 mg
Sodium 59 mg
Carbohydrates 23 g
Fiber 2 g
Sugars 3 g
Protein 5 g
Calcium 46 mg
Potassium 116 mg
Dietary Exchanges:
1½ starch, ½ fat

CINNAMON-SUGAR TOPPING

Calories 150
Total Fat 3.5 g
Saturated Fat 0.5 g
Trans Fat 0.0 g
Polyunsaturated Fat 0.5 g
Monounsaturated Fat 2.0 g
Cholesterol 16 mg
Sodium 59 mg
Carbohydrates 27 g
Fiber 2 g
Sugars 7 g
Protein 5 g
Calcium 35 mg
Potassium 106 mg
Dietary Exchanges:
2 starch

SODIUM SMARTS: In general, pretzels—unless they're unsalted—are high in sodium because salt is not only in the dough but also on it, for the salty topping. The salted variety can contain about 500 mg of sodium per serving. A medium soft pretzel can have more than 900 mg—60 percent of the American Heart Association's daily sodium recommendation of 1,500 mg! Instead, enjoy our recipe for Hot Soft Pretzels with your choice of toppings for about 60 mg of sodium per serving.

Three-Way Popcorn

A warm and crunchy popcorn treat always brings a smile, especially when you know it can satisfy your cravings for sweet *or* savory. This recipe provides three palate-pleasing options, all low in sodium.

SERVES 4
2 cups per serving

- **1 tablespoon canola or corn oil (for Sweet Cinnamon Seasoning or Lemon-Herb Seasoning)**

  or

- **1 tablespoon olive oil (extra virgin preferred) (for Parmesan-Pepper Seasoning)**
- **¼ cup popcorn kernels**

SWEET CINNAMON SEASONING

- **2 tablespoons sugar**
- **½ teaspoon ground cinnamon**
- **⅛ teaspoon ground nutmeg**
- **Butter-flavor cooking spray**

LEMON-HERB SEASONING

- **1 tablespoon grated lemon zest**
- **½ teaspoon dried oregano, crumbled**
- **¼ teaspoon garlic powder**
- **¼ teaspoon dried rosemary, crushed**
- **Olive oil cooking spray or butter-flavor cooking spray**

CONTINUED

1. If cooking on the stovetop, in a large saucepan, heat the oil over medium heat, swirling to coat the bottom. Stir in the popcorn kernels. Cover the pan, leaving the lid slightly ajar. Cook until the popping stops (no need to shake the pan), about 2 minutes from when the popcorn begins to pop. Remove the pan from the heat. Alternatively, if using a popcorn popper, follow the manufacturer's directions.

2. Meanwhile, for the seasoning mixture of your choice, put the ingredients except the cooking spray in a small bowl, stirring to combine. Set aside.

3. Lightly spray the popcorn with cooking spray. Sprinkle with the seasoning mixture, tossing until well blended. Serve immediately for peak flavor and texture.

SODIUM SMARTS: For a topping with a kick, try sprinkling your popped popcorn with a salt-free jerk seasoning blend (sometimes called Jamaican jerk seasoning). If you can't find it in stores or want only a small amount, make your own no-sodium version. In a small bowl, stir together ½ teaspoon ground cumin, ¼ teaspoon ground allspice, and ¼ teaspoon ground cinnamon, plus black pepper and/or cayenne to taste.

PARMESAN-PEPPER SEASONING

- 2 tablespoons shredded or grated Parmesan cheese
- ¼ to ½ teaspoon pepper (coarsely ground preferred)
- ¼ teaspoon dried dillweed, crumbled (optional)
- Olive oil cooking spray

PER SERVING

WITH SWEET CINNAMON SEASONING

Calories 118
Total Fat 4.0 g
Saturated Fat 0.5 g
Trans Fat 0.0 g
Polyunsaturated Fat 1.5 g
Monounsaturated Fat 2.5 g
Cholesterol 0 mg
Sodium 1 mg
Carbohydrates 19 g
Fiber 2 g
Sugars 7 g
Protein 2 g
Calcium 4 mg
Potassium 47 mg
Dietary Exchanges:
1 starch, 1 fat

WITH LEMON-HERB SEASONING

Calories 95
Total Fat 4.0 g
Saturated Fat 0.0 g
Trans Fat 0.0 g
Polyunsaturated Fat 1.5 g
Monounsaturated Fat 2.5 g
Cholesterol 0 mg
Sodium 1 mg
Carbohydrates 13 g
Fiber 2 g
Sugars 0 g
Protein 2 g
Calcium 6 mg
Potassium 54 mg
Dietary Exchanges:
1 starch, 1 fat

WITH PARMESAN-PEPPER SEASONING

Calories 103
Total Fat 5.0 g
Saturated Fat 1.0 g
Trans Fat 0.0 g
Polyunsaturated Fat 1.0 g
Monounsaturated Fat 3.0 g
Cholesterol 2 mg
Sodium 44 mg
Carbohydrates 12 g
Fiber 2 g
Sugars 0 g
Protein 3 g
Calcium 33 mg
Potassium 51 mg
Dietary Exchanges:
1 starch, 1 fat

Granola Mini Bars

All snacks should have the variety of flavors that this one does. Every bite is full of toasted nuttiness and concentrated fruitiness.

SERVES 16
one 2-inch square per serving

- **Cooking spray**
- **2 cups bite-size whole-wheat cereal squares (lowest sodium available)**
- **1 cup broken unsalted pretzels (1-inch pieces)**
- **½ cup white whole-wheat flour**
- **½ cup sugar**
- **½ cup unsalted shelled pistachios**
- **½ cup sweetened dried cranberries**
- **2 large egg whites**
- **⅓ cup canola or corn oil**
- **¼ cup sliced almonds or unsalted shelled sunflower seeds**
- **¼ cup mini chocolate chips**
- **2 teaspoons grated orange zest**
- **1 teaspoon ground cinnamon**
- **⅛ teaspoon salt**

1. Preheat the oven to 325°F. Line the bottom and sides of an 8-inch square baking pan with aluminum foil. Lightly spray the foil with cooking spray.

2. In a large bowl, stir together all the ingredients. Transfer the granola to the pan. Using your fingertips, press it into the pan so the ingredients adhere to each other, then flatten it.

3. Bake for 35 minutes, or until lightly browned. Transfer the pan to a cooling rack. Let the granola cool completely, about 2 hours.

4. Place a cutting board over the pan. Turn the pan over. Discard the foil. Using a serrated knife, carefully cut the large square into 16 small squares.

5. Store leftovers in an airtight container at room temperature for up to one week.

PER SERVING
Calories 179
Total Fat 8.5 g
Saturated Fat 1.0 g
Trans Fat 0.0 g
Polyunsaturated Fat 2.0 g
Monounsaturated Fat 4.5 g
Cholesterol 0 mg
Sodium 86 mg
Carbohydrates 25 g
Fiber 2 g
Sugars 12 g
Protein 3 g
Calcium 29 mg
Potassium 116 mg
Dietary Exchanges:
1½ other carbohydrate, 2 fat

Italian-Style Tortilla Chips

These chips are delicious on their own or with our Fresh Tomato-Tomatillo Salsa (page 210). You can pack them in lunch boxes or break them up to sprinkle on soups instead of salty crackers.

SERVES 10
8 chips per serving

- **1 teaspoon garlic powder**
- **1 teaspoon dried oregano, crumbled**
- **½ teaspoon dried thyme, crumbled**
- **½ teaspoon pepper (coarsely ground preferred)**
- **¼ teaspoon dried rosemary, crushed**
- **10 6-inch corn tortillas**
- **1 tablespoon canola or corn oil**

1. Preheat the oven to 350°F.

2. In a small bowl, stir together the garlic powder, oregano, thyme, pepper, and rosemary. Set aside.

3. Stack the tortillas on a cutting board. Cut the stack into 8 triangles (80 wedges total). Arrange the triangles in a single layer on each of two large baking sheets.

4. Drizzle the chips with the oil. Sprinkle with the garlic powder mixture.

5. Bake for 10 to 11 minutes, or until the chips are light brown and beginning to crisp. Transfer the baking sheets to cooling racks. Let cool completely, about 15 minutes (as the chips cool, they will become crisper).

6. Store in an airtight container for up to one week. If you don't need so many chips within a week, make only half the recipe.

PER SERVING
Calories 46
Total Fat 2.0 g
Saturated Fat 0.0 g
Trans Fat 0.0 g
Polyunsaturated Fat 0.5 g
Monounsaturated Fat 1.0 g
Cholesterol 0 mg
Sodium 23 mg
Carbohydrates 7 g
Fiber 1 g
Sugars 0 g
Protein 1 g
Calcium 28 mg
Potassium 30 mg
Dietary Exchanges:
½ starch

Herbed Veggie Chips

The next time you get the munchies, bake a batch of these thin, crisp veggie chips. They contain 2 grams of healthful fiber in every serving and get so much flavor from herbs and spices that only a little salt is needed. The same tasty combination of seasonings is used to make the Italian-Style Tortilla Chips (page 201).

SERVES 5
½ cup per serving

- Cooking spray
- 1 teaspoon garlic powder
- 1 teaspoon dried oregano, crumbled
- ½ teaspoon dried thyme, crumbled
- ½ teaspoon pepper (coarsely ground preferred)
- ¼ teaspoon dried rosemary, crushed
- 6 ounces fingerling potatoes (4 or 5 large)
- 3 ounces carrots (1 or 2 medium, no more than 1-inch diameter)
- 3 ounces parsnips (1 or 2 medium, no more than 1-inch diameter)
- 1 tablespoon canola or corn oil
- ¼ teaspoon salt

1. Preheat the oven to 400°F. Lightly spray two large baking sheets with cooking spray. Set aside.

2. In a small bowl, stir together the garlic powder, oregano, thyme, pepper, and rosemary. Set aside.

3. Using the slicing blade of a food processor or a mandolin or slicing by hand, slice the potatoes, carrots, and parsnips as thin as possible, being sure the slices are less than ⅛ inch thick and keeping the potatoes separate. Place the potatoes on one baking sheet and the carrots and parsnips on the other.

4. Drizzle the potatoes with half the oil, stirring to coat. Arrange in a single layer. Sprinkle with half the garlic powder mixture. Repeat the process with the carrots and parsnips. Set them aside.

5. Bake the potatoes for 4 minutes. Leaving the potatoes in the oven, put the carrots and parsnips on a separate oven rack. Bake for 6 minutes. Stir the vegetables on both baking sheets. Bake for 5 to 6 minutes, or until most of the slices begin to brown on the edges. Transfer the baking sheets to cooling racks.

6. Sprinkle the chips with the salt. Don't stir. Let the chips cool slightly, about 5 minutes. Carefully transfer to a serving plate or large shallow bowl (the chips will be fragile). Serve immediately for peak flavor and texture.

PER SERVING

Calories 73
Total Fat 3.0 g
 Saturated Fat 0.0 g
 Trans Fat 0.0 g
 Polyunsaturated Fat 1.0 g
 Monounsaturated Fat 2.0 g
Cholesterol 0 mg
Sodium 136 mg
Carbohydrates 11 g
 Fiber 2 g
 Sugars 2 g
Protein 1 g
Calcium 22 mg
Potassium 290 mg
Dietary Exchanges:
½ starch, ½ fat

White Bean, Kalamata, and Basil Hummus

Packed with plenty of fresh basil, plus garlic and kalamata olives, this hummus pops with flavor. It uses white beans instead of chickpeas for a twist and gets a color boost from its toppings. Use any of the traditional vegetables—carrots, broccoli, or cauliflower—for dipping, or try some unusual choices, such as sugar snap peas or pieces of fennel.

SERVES 6
¼ cup per serving

HUMMUS

- 1 15.5-ounce can no-salt-added navy beans, rinsed and drained
- ½ cup chopped fresh basil
- ¼ cup fat-free plain yogurt (Greek preferred)
- 12 kalamata olives, pitted
- 2 tablespoons fresh lemon juice
- 1 tablespoon olive oil (extra virgin preferred)
- 1 tablespoon red wine vinegar
- 2 medium garlic cloves
- ¼ teaspoon ground cumin

TOPPINGS

- 2 to 3 tablespoons chopped fresh basil
- 2 tablespoons chopped roasted red bell pepper, drained if bottled
- 1 tablespoon olive oil (extra virgin preferred)

1. In a food processor or blender, process the hummus ingredients until smooth. Spoon into a shallow serving dish.

2. Sprinkle the hummus with the remaining 2 to 3 tablespoons basil and the roasted pepper. Drizzle with the remaining 1 tablespoon oil.

3. To serve the hummus up to two days after preparing, refrigerate it in an airtight container. Just before serving time, prepare the toppings and proceed as directed.

SODIUM SMARTS: With only 11 mg of sodium per teaspoon, this homemade hummus also can be a flavorful sodium-saving replacement for sandwich spreads. Lightly spread it on low-sodium bread, such as our Whole-Grain and Honey Bread (page 138), and wraps instead of using yellow mustard (about 45 mg per teaspoon) or light mayonnaise (about 40 mg per teaspoon).

PER SERVING

Calories 132	Carbohydrates 13 g
Total Fat 6.5 g	Fiber 3 g
Saturated Fat 1.0 g	Sugars 3 g
Trans Fat 0.0 g	Protein 5 g
Polyunsaturated Fat 0.5 g	Calcium 54 mg
Monounsaturated Fat 5.0 g	Potassium 309 mg
Cholesterol 0 mg	Dietary Exchanges:
Sodium 132 mg	1 starch, 1 fat

Nutty Cereal-and-Seeds Snack Mix

Baking the grains, nuts, and seeds in this snack mix brings out their flavors, which complement the sweetness of the cranberries and the tanginess of the orange zest. Use the optional smoked paprika if you want to add a deep, aromatic flavor.

SERVES 12
⅓ cup per serving

- 2 cups bite-size whole-wheat cereal squares (lowest sodium available)
- ½ cup unsalted shelled pistachios
- 2 ounces unsalted pretzels, broken into 1-inch pieces
- 2 ounces unsalted pumpkin seeds in shells
- 2 tablespoons canola or corn oil
- Cooking spray
- ½ cup sweetened dried cranberries
- 2 teaspoons grated orange zest
- 2 teaspoons smoked paprika (optional)
- 1 teaspoon ground cinnamon

1. Preheat the oven to 300°F.

2. In a large bowl, stir together the cereal squares, pistachios, pretzels, and pumpkin seeds. Drizzle with the oil. Toss gently to coat. Spread in a single layer on a large rimmed baking sheet.

3. Bake for 16 minutes, stirring once halfway through. Transfer to a cooling rack.

4. Lightly spray the mixture with cooking spray. Sprinkle with the remaining ingredients. Toss gently. Let cool for 10 minutes to become crisp.

5. Let leftover trail mix cool completely, at least 1 hour (in addition to the 10 minutes). Store in an airtight container at room temperature for up to two weeks.

SODIUM SMARTS: Many ready-to-eat cereals are loaded with not only sugar but also sodium—as much as 360 mg in 1 cup! Buy the brand with the lowest sodium, or mix your brand with one that has little or no sodium. Or supplement a small amount of cereal with fresh fruit.

PER SERVING

Calories 151
Total Fat 7.5 g
Saturated Fat 1.0 g
Trans Fat 0.0 g
Polyunsaturated Fat 2.5 g
Monounsaturated Fat 3.5 g
Cholesterol 0 mg
Sodium 72 mg
Carbohydrates 19 g
Fiber 3 g
Sugars 6 g
Protein 4 g
Calcium 32 mg
Potassium 150 mg
Dietary Exchanges: 1½ starch, 1 fat

SAUCES, GRAVIES, CONDIMENTS, AND SEASONINGS

Do you think of seasonings as "free" foods? They may be free in calories and fats, but they may not be sodium free. Other food complements, such as condiments, sauces, and gravies, usually are loaded with sodium, too. Most of the processed foods in these categories contain high levels of sodium per serving, and some that might not even seem especially high are among the sneakiest sources. Did you know that 1 tablespoon of soy sauce has, on average, about 1,000 mg of sodium, or that just a few green olives can easily contain more than a third of the daily sodium recommendation? Look at the chart on pages 207 and 208 for other surprising sources.

TRY THESE LOWER-SODIUM RECIPES:

- Fresh Tomato-Tomatillo Salsa (page 210)
- Smoky Sweet Barbecue Sauce (page 211)
- Brown Gravy (page 212)
- Alfredo Sauce (page 213)
- Spicy-Sweet Citrus-Cilantro Marinade (page 214)
- Mamma Mia Marinara (page 215)

SPOTLIGHT ON: Ketchup and Mustard

Just 1 tablespoon of either of these condiments can pack about 200 mg of sodium. If you like to slather your hot dog or hamburger with one (or even both) of these popular toppers, you could be eating about 400 mg of sodium—more than 25 percent of the recommended daily sodium intake, in condiments alone!

SODIUM IN SELECTED SAUCES, GRAVIES, CONDIMENTS, AND SEASONINGS

FOOD	SODIUM (MG)*
marinara sauce, ½ cup	220–780
Mamma Mia Marinara (page 215), ½ cup	15
Alfredo sauce, ¼ cup	320–490
Alfredo Sauce (page 213), ¼ cup	220
spaghetti sauce with mushrooms, ½ cup	480–630
spaghetti sauce with roasted garlic, ½ cup	220–780
spaghetti sauce with spinach and cheese, ½ cup	460
salsa, ¼ cup	230–500
Fresh Tomato-Tomatillo Salsa (page 210), ¼ cup	60
marinade, 1 tbsp	340–610
Spicy-Sweet Citrus-Cilantro Marinade (page 214), ½ cup	0
pesto, ¼ cup	475–720
barbecue sauce, 2 tbsp	265–450
Smoky Sweet Barbecue Sauce (page 211), ¼ cup	145
steak sauce, 2 tbsp	380–730
Worcestershire sauce, 1 tbsp	165–180
tomato sauce, ¼ cup	280–410
tomato sauce, no salt added, ¼ cup	5–20
tomato paste, 2 tbsp	105–290
tomato paste, no salt added, 2 tbsp	10–30
soy sauce, 1 tbsp	920–1,315
soy sauce, light, 1 tbsp	505–575
teriyaki sauce, 1 tbsp	390–690
teriyaki sauce, light, 1 tbsp	320–440
oyster sauce, 1 tbsp	490–900
cocktail sauce, 1 tbsp	100–230
Cocktail Sauce (page 172), 1 tbsp	85
tartar sauce, 1 tbsp	75–150

***Sodium values have been rounded to the nearest 5 mg.**

CONTINUED

FOOD	SODIUM (MG)*
brown gravy mix, prepared, 2 tbsp	150–190
Brown Gravy (page 212), 2 tbsp	120
turkey gravy, 2 tbsp	145–170
ketchup, 1 tbsp	160–210
ketchup, no-salt-added, 1 tbsp	0–5
mustard, yellow, 1 tbsp	80–170
mustard, Dijon, 1 tbsp	120–360
mustard, honey, 1 tbsp	15–125
capers, 1 tbsp	255–420
olives, black, 1 oz	210–245
olives, green, 1 oz	440–585
pickles, dill, 1 oz	250–305
mayonnaise, 1 tbsp	50–90
mayonnaise, light, 1 tbsp	100–120
pickle relish, dill, 1 tbsp	230–270
pickle relish, sweet, 1 tbsp	95–125
peanut butter, 2 tbsp	120–150
peanut butter, low-sodium, 2 tbsp	0–65
bacon bits, 1 tbsp	80–220
meat tenderizer, ¼ tsp	300–420
garlic salt, ¼ tsp	240
garlic powder, ¼ tsp	0
onion salt, ¼ tsp	170–450
onion powder, ¼ tsp	0
celery salt, ¼ tsp	250
celery flakes, ¼ tsp	5
table salt, ¼ tsp	580
fresh or dried herbs, such as basil, oregano, parsley, and cilantro, and spices, 1 tbsp	0

***Sodium values have been rounded to the nearest 5 mg.**

SODIUM-SAVING SOLUTIONS

- Herbs and spices are great for enhancing flavor without adding sodium, but watch out for seasoning salts, such as garlic, onion, and celery. Instead use garlic powder, onion powder, and celery flakes. Also, check the spice aisle for different varieties of salt-free seasonings.
- Watch out for seasonings that contain monosodium glutamate (MSG), which, as its full name indicates, is sodium heavy.
- To get the most flavor benefit from dried herbs and spices, store them in airtight containers in a cool, dark place. Dried herbs and spices have a shelf life of about six months. After that, they may lose their potency and thus their potential to add flavor to your food. Label the containers with the date you purchase the herbs and spices so you know when it's time to replace them.
- Fresh herbs contain no sodium and impart great flavor to a dish. Since they aren't concentrated like their dried counterparts, you'll need to use three times as much of the fresh herb as you would of the dried.
- Fresh herbs do not last long in the refrigerator, so wash and dry them, then freeze them, whole or chopped, in labeled airtight bags. You don't need to defrost frozen herbs before using them.
- In place of a saltshaker, keep shakers with your favorite dried herbs and spices, such as garlic powder or cayenne, on the table.
- Scan the grocery store shelves for no-salt-added, reduced-sodium, and light seasoning products, and find the lowest-sodium options.
- Avoid regular bouillon cubes or crystals, or use them sparingly.
- Generally, the sweeter mustards, such as honey mustard, are lower in sodium than other mustards, such as yellow and Dijon.
- Most bottled, jarred, or canned sauces are high in sodium. Read the nutrition facts panels and choose the lowest-sodium varieties.
- Soy, fish, and teriyaki sauces and tamari are loaded with sodium, so choose the lowest-sodium products and use them sparingly or replace them with low-salt options. Spice up a stir-fry with fresh garlic, ginger root, chiles, plain rice vinegar, and fresh lime juice.
- Miso, or fermented soy paste, is available in many varieties, each with a different flavor and degree of saltiness. Look for the lighter-colored varieties, such as chickpea miso, which usually are lower in salt content than the darker ones.

Fresh Tomato-Tomatillo Salsa

For red salsa with a difference, do as many authentic Mexican restaurants do—use green tomatillos along with the usual red tomatoes. Try this salsa with Italian-Style Tortilla Chips (page 201), or Herbed Veggie Chips (page 202), use it to dress Mexican-style salads, or top baked potatoes or scrambled eggs with it.

SERVES 10
¼ cup per serving

2 cups chopped tomatoes (about 2 medium)
¼ cup diced red onion
⅓ cup snipped fresh cilantro
½ medium poblano chile, seeds and ribs discarded, diced, or 1 medium fresh jalapeño, seeds and ribs discarded, diced
1½ tablespoons fresh lime juice
1½ tablespoons cider vinegar
½ cup finely chopped tomatillo (about 1 medium, husk discarded)
¼ teaspoon salt

1. In a small bowl, stir together all the ingredients.

2. Serve at room temperature or cover and refrigerate until needed. For peak flavor and texture, serve within 12 hours.

SODIUM SMARTS: Remember that jarred salsas often are big offenders when it comes to high sodium content. Just ¼ cup of salsa can contain, on average, 365 mg of sodium—six times more than the same amount of our salsa!

PER SERVING
Calories 12
Total Fat 0.0 g
Saturated Fat 0.0 g
Trans Fat 0.0 g
Polyunsaturated Fat 0.0 g
Monounsaturated Fat 0.0 g
Cholesterol 0 mg
Sodium 61 mg
Carbohydrates 3 g
Fiber 1 g
Sugars 1 g
Protein 1 g
Calcium 6 mg
Potassium 118 mg
Dietary Exchanges: Free

Smoky Sweet Barbecue Sauce

Use this savory sauce recipe so you can eat those grilled entrées you love and still keep your sodium intake under control.

SERVES 5
¼ cup per serving

- 2 teaspoons canola or corn oil
- ½ cup chopped onion
- 1 8-ounce can no-salt-added tomato sauce
- ¼ cup no-salt-added tomato paste
- ¼ cup water
- 2 tablespoons firmly packed dark brown sugar
- 2 tablespoons honey
- 1 tablespoon balsamic vinegar
- 1½ to 2 teaspoons liquid smoke (lowest sodium available)
- 1 teaspoon Worcestershire sauce (lowest sodium available)
- ¼ teaspoon ground cumin
- ¼ teaspoon salt
- ⅛ teaspoon cayenne
- 2 teaspoons grated orange zest

1. In a medium saucepan, heat the oil over medium heat, swirling to coat the bottom. Cook the onion for 4 minutes, stirring frequently.

2. Stir in the remaining ingredients except the orange zest. Bring to a boil, still over medium heat. Reduce the heat and simmer for 20 minutes, or until the sauce has thickened slightly and the onion is very soft. Remove from the heat. Stir in the orange zest. Let cool completely, about 1 hour, so the sauce thickens and the flavors blend.

3. Refrigerate leftovers in an airtight container for up to one week or freeze them in an airtight freezer container for up to six months.

SODIUM SMARTS: You may know that bottled barbecue sauce is full of sugar, but did you realize that it's also loaded with sodium? Depending on the flavor and brand, you'll most likely get at least 530 mg, more than one-third of the recommended daily sodium allowance, in just ¼ cup. This version checks in with less than 150 mg for the same amount.

PER SERVING

Calories 104	Carbohydrates 21 g
Total Fat 2.0 g	Fiber 2 g
Saturated Fat 0.0 g	Sugars 18 g
Trans Fat 0.0 g	Protein 1 g
Polyunsaturated Fat 0.5 g	Calcium 23 mg
Monounsaturated Fat 1.0 g	Potassium 346 mg
Cholesterol 0 mg	Dietary Exchanges:
Sodium 146 mg	1 other carbohydrate, ½ fat

Brown Gravy

Brown gravies are known for their rich flavor, but the ones in jars or from packets tend to be sodium heavy. This recipe calls for cooking the flour first and using instant coffee granules to provide rich, complex taste but nowhere near that overabundance of sodium.

SERVES 6
2 tablespoons per serving

- **1½ tablespoons all-purpose flour**
- **1½ tablespoons canola or corn oil**
- **1½ tablespoons light tub margarine**
- **1 cup water**
- **1 packet (1 teaspoon) salt-free instant beef bouillon**
- **½ teaspoon instant coffee granules (espresso preferred)**
- **½ to 1 teaspoon Worcestershire sauce (lowest sodium available)**
- **¼ teaspoon salt**

1. Heat a medium nonstick skillet over medium heat for about 2 minutes, or until hot. Cook the flour for 3 minutes, or until beginning to lightly brown, stirring constantly.

2. Whisk in the oil and margarine until the margarine is melted.

3. Gradually whisk in the water. Whisk in the remaining ingredients. Cook for 3 minutes, or until the gravy is thickened, whisking constantly.

SODIUM SMARTS: Salt-free powdered chicken and beef bouillon are available in convenient 1-teaspoon packets. Containing 0 to 5 mg of sodium, they are without question a much healthier choice than the equivalent chicken bouillon cubes, which range from 960 to 1,150 mg of sodium per cube, and beef cubes, which range from 610 to 1,005 mg.

PER SERVING

Calories 50
Total Fat 4.5 g
Saturated Fat 0.5 g
Trans Fat 0.0 g
Polyunsaturated Fat 1.0 g
Monounsaturated Fat 3.0 g
Cholesterol 0 mg
Sodium 122 mg
Carbohydrates 2 g
Fiber 0 g
Sugars 0 g
Protein 0 g
Calcium 99 mg
Potassium 2 mg
Dietary Exchanges: 1 fat

Alfredo Sauce

This easy-to-make sauce, much lower in sodium than you're likely to find in Italian restaurants, is creamy, cheesy, and garlicky. Because of its richness, just a little of the sauce goes a long, long way. Spoon it over side servings of whole-grain pastas or steamed vegetables, or use it to dress up lightly seasoned chicken breasts or fish fillets.

SERVES 4
¼ cup per serving

- 1 cup fat-free milk
- 1 tablespoon all-purpose flour
- 2 tablespoons light tub cream cheese
- 2 medium garlic cloves, minced
- ¼ cup shredded or grated Parmesan cheese
- ⅛ teaspoon salt

In a medium saucepan, whisk together the milk and flour. Whisk in the cream cheese and garlic. Cook over medium-high heat for 3 to 4 minutes, or until thickened, whisking constantly. Whisk in the Parmesan and salt. Remove from the heat.

PER SERVING
Calories 68
Total Fat 2.5 g
Saturated Fat 1.5 g
Trans Fat 0.0 g
Polyunsaturated Fat 0.0 g
Monounsaturated Fat 1.0 g
Cholesterol 10 mg
Sodium 218 mg
Carbohydrates 6 g
Fiber 0 g
Sugars 4 g
Protein 5 g
Calcium 165 mg
Potassium 122 mg
Dietary Exchanges: 1 fat

Spicy-Sweet Citrus-Cilantro Marinade

Jazz up your meal by marinating the meat, seafood, or poultry in this tangy marinade.

MAKES ½ CUP
enough for 1 to 1½ pounds of seafood, poultry, or meat

- ¼ cup fresh lime juice
- 2 tablespoons snipped fresh cilantro
- 2 tablespoons water
- 1 tablespoon thinly sliced green onions
- 1 tablespoon honey
- 2 medium garlic cloves, minced
- 1 teaspoon plain rice vinegar
- 1 teaspoon olive oil
- ½ teaspoon crushed red pepper flakes

1. In a small bowl, whisk together all the ingredients.

2. Refrigerate for up to two days in an airtight container.

SODIUM SMARTS: Homemade marinades are the healthy way to go, since bottled varieties are notoriously high in sodium, with some containing more than 600 mg per tablespoon. Red wine vinegar, fresh lemon juice, and fresh orange juice are excellent sodium-free meat and poultry tenderizers.

PER SERVING
Calories 17
Total Fat 0.5 g
Saturated Fat 0.0 g
Trans Fat 0.0 g
Polyunsaturated Fat 0.0 g
Monounsaturated Fat 0.0 g
Cholesterol 0 mg
Sodium 0 mg
Carbohydrates 2 g
Fiber 0 g
Sugars 1 g
Protein 0 g
Calcium 0 mg
Potassium 0 mg
Dietary Exchanges: Free

Mamma Mia Marinara

Lots of garlic plus fresh basil, dried herbes de Provence (a standout seasoning blend of herbs from southern France), sugar, and a blast of red pepper flakes add flavor without sodium to this robust tomato sauce. Use it to top all your favorite pasta dishes—and homemade pizzas (see Pizza Dough on page 135).

SERVES 6
½ cup per serving

- 4 large or very large garlic cloves, minced
- 1 tablespoon olive oil
- 1 28-ounce can no-salt-added crushed tomatoes, undrained
- 1 tablespoon chopped fresh basil
- 1 teaspoon dried herbes de Provence, crumbled
- 1 teaspoon sugar
- ¼ to ½ teaspoon crushed red pepper flakes

1. In a medium saucepan, cook the garlic and oil for 2 to 3 minutes over medium heat, stirring frequently. Watch carefully so the garlic doesn't brown.

2. Stir in the remaining ingredients. Increase the heat to medium high and bring to a boil. Reduce the heat and simmer, covered, for 1 hour, or until the sauce is the desired consistency, stirring occasionally.

3. Refrigerate leftover sauce in an airtight container for up to five days or freeze it in an airtight freezer container for up to six months.

SODIUM SMARTS: One-half cup of bottled spaghetti sauce can easily hit you with about a third—or more—of our daily sodium recommendation. Control your sodium intake with this fresh-tasting sauce that has only 16 mg in the same size serving.

PER SERVING

Calories 56	Carbohydrates 8 g
Total Fat 2.5 g	Fiber 1 g
Saturated Fat 0.5 g	Sugars 5 g
Trans Fat 0.0 g	Protein 1 g
Polyunsaturated Fat 0.0 g	Calcium 25 mg
Monounsaturated Fat 1.5 g	Potassium 10 mg
Cholesterol 0 mg	Dietary Exchanges:
Sodium 16 mg	2 vegetable, ½ fat

SALADS AND SALAD DRESSINGS

When you're deciding what to eat, do you assume a salad is a wise food choice? Maybe it is, but maybe it isn't. What is in that salad and how it is dressed determine how nutritious it really is. You may have a salad full of good-for-you ingredients, but if they are soaked in sodium-laden salad dressings and topped with croutons, bacon bits, and cheese—all sodium traps—the health value of that salad is greatly diminished.

TRY THESE LOWER-SODIUM SALAD AND DRESSING RECIPES:

- Gazpacho Pasta Salad (page 219)
- Retro Marinated Bean Salad (page 220)
- Garlic-Dill Potato Salad (page 221)
- Curried Tuna Salad with Almonds (page 222)
- Coleslaw with Ginger and Celery Seeds (page 223)
- Ranch-Style Dressing with Green Onions (page 224)
- Basil-Garlic Italian Dressing (page 225)
- Thousand Island Dressing (page 226)

SPOTLIGHT ON: Salad Dressings Consumers' health concerns about salad dressings seem to focus on the fat and calories they contain, but sodium needs to be another area of attention. Most of the salad dressings on supermarket shelves have at least 200 mg of sodium in a 2-tablespoon serving, with others close to 400 mg—and even more. If you are heavy-handed with the dressing, you can easily consume double those amounts—in the dressing alone.

SODIUM IN SELECTED SALADS AND SALAD DRESSINGS

FOOD	SODIUM (MG)*
potato salad, 4 oz	545
Garlic-Dill Potato Salad (page 221), ½ cup	105
coleslaw, 4 oz	240
Coleslaw with Ginger and Celery Seeds (page 223), ½ cup	50
macaroni salad, 4 oz	600
pasta salad, 4 oz	410–605
Gazpacho Pasta Salad (page 219), 1½ cups	235
bean salad, 4 oz	340–600
Retro Marinated Bean Salad (page 220), ½ cup	150
tuna salad, 4 oz	455–660
Curried Tuna Salad with Almonds (page 222), ⅔ cup	160
Caesar dressing, 2 tbsp	170–440
French dressing, 2 tbsp	260–600
French dressing, fat-free, 2 tbsp	255–300
Italian dressing, 2 tbsp	300–510
Italian dressing, fat-free, 2 tbsp	280–380
Basil-Garlic Italian Dressing (page 225), 2 tbsp	145
blue cheese dressing, 2 tbsp	170–310
ranch dressing, 2 tbsp	150–370
ranch dressing, fat-free, 2 tbsp	250–330
ranch dressing, mix, 1 tsp	315–555
Ranch-Style Dressing with Green Onions (page 224), 2 tbsp	150
Thousand Island dressing, 2 tbsp	210–310
Thousand Island dressing, fat-free, 2 tbsp	280–320
Thousand Island Dressing (page 226), 2 tbsp	115
vinegar, oil, and fresh herbs, 2 tbsp	0

***Sodium values have been rounded to the nearest 5 mg.**

SODIUM-SAVING SOLUTIONS

- Be mindful that the fat-free varieties of salad dressings often have more sodium than their full-fat or low-fat counterparts, so don't be misled into thinking that the fat-free choices are always the best.
- Avoid salad dressings that are made with dried mixes, which are loaded with sodium, and use bottled salad dressings sparingly since they usually are high in sodium.
- If you aren't paying much attention when you pour dressing onto a salad, it's easy to go overboard. Focus on adding no more than 2 tablespoons, especially if you're using a commercial salad dressing. The sodium, calories, and fat quickly add up, even before you count whatever food you are topping.
- A good way to monitor how much salad dressing you eat is to serve 2 tablespoons of the dressing on the side and lightly dip each bite of food into it. You'll be surprised at how little dressing it really takes to provide the flavor you are used to.
- Although spinach has more naturally occurring sodium than most other vegetables (see "Vegetables and Fruits"), it is well worth enjoying in your salads because it is full of beneficial minerals and vitamins.
- Add your favorite fresh herbs to your salad greens for a flavor boost.
- Add pizzazz to an ordinary salad with ingredients that have a bit of a bite, including radishes, red onion, fresh jalapeños, pico de gallo (diced onion, tomatoes, and jalapeño), and red pepper flakes.
- Seasoned croutons can bring down the health factor of your salad because they are sodium-rich. If you want to add crunch to your salad, try sprinkling it with dry-roasted unsalted nuts, unsalted sunflower seeds, or a few crumbled Italian-Style Tortilla Chips or Herbed Veggie Chips (see recipes on pages 201 and 202).
- Avoid or limit adding salty ingredients, including cheeses, processed meats, and condiments such as bacon bits, to your salad. They add up quickly and can turn an otherwise healthy salad into a less healthy, high-sodium nightmare.
- A basic, easy, and healthy salt-free salad dressing is a mixture of two or three parts olive oil to one part vinegar. Flavor the dressing by adding fresh herbs or salt-free seasoning blends, such as lemon pepper, and trying different vinegars or substituting fresh citrus juice.

Gazpacho Pasta Salad

The low-sodium version of either spicy mixed-vegetable juice or Bloody Mary mix is the base for the fast dressing that goes into this garden-fresh entrée salad.

SERVES 6
1½ cups per serving

- 8 ounces dried whole-grain fusilli or rotini (about 3 cups)
- 2 ounces spinach, chopped (about 2 cups)
- 1 small cucumber, quartered lengthwise and sliced crosswise (about 1 cup)
- 4 ounces cherry or grape tomatoes, halved (about 1 cup)
- 1 cup cooked shelled edamame (green soybeans)
- 1 small green or red bell pepper, chopped
- ⅓ cup finely chopped red onion
- ¼ cup snipped fresh parsley
- ¾ cup low-sodium spicy mixed-vegetable juice or low-sodium Bloody Mary mix
- 3 tablespoons fresh lime juice
- 1 medium garlic clove, minced
- 1 medium avocado, chopped
- Red hot-pepper sauce (optional)

1. Prepare the pasta using the package directions, omitting the salt. Drain in a colander. Run under cold water to stop the cooking process and cool quickly. Drain well. Transfer to a large bowl.

2. Add the spinach, cucumber, tomatoes, edamame, bell pepper, onion, and parsley, tossing to combine.

3. In a small bowl, stir together the vegetable juice, lime juice, and garlic. Pour into the pasta mixture, tossing to coat. Gently stir in the avocado. Cover and refrigerate for 1 to 4 hours before serving. Serve with the hot-pepper sauce to sprinkle on top.

SODIUM SMARTS: For 8 ounces of spicy mixed-vegetable juice, the regular variety can contain 600 mg or more of sodium. We call for the low-sodium product, which for the equivalent amount has less than one-third the sodium. Be sure to look for the lowest-sodium Bloody Mary mix you can find if you opt for that ingredient. Most regular mixes contain over 1,000 mg of sodium in 8 ounces.

PER SERVING

Calories 247
Total Fat 7.0 g
Saturated Fat 1.0 g
Trans Fat 0.0 g
Polyunsaturated Fat 1.5 g
Monounsaturated Fat 4.0 g
Cholesterol 0 mg
Sodium 233 mg
Carbohydrates 40 g
Fiber 8 g
Sugars 5 g
Protein 11 g
Calcium 58 mg
Potassium 667 mg
Dietary Exchanges: 2 starch, 2 vegetable, 1 fat

Retro Marinated Bean Salad

This brightly colored dish is inviting and so easy to make. If you're having friends over for a barbecue, double all the ingredients for a simple side that goes well with beef or chicken. To make up to two days ahead, refrigerate the bean mixture and dressing in separate containers, then toss together when you're ready to serve.

SERVES 6
½ cup per serving

SALAD

- ½ 15.5-ounce can no-salt-added kidney beans or no-salt-added small red beans, rinsed and drained
- ½ 15.5-ounce can no-salt-added black beans, rinsed and drained
- ½ 14.5-ounce can no-salt-added cut green beans, rinsed and drained
- ½ cup chopped red or yellow onion
- ½ medium yellow bell pepper, chopped

DRESSING

- 3 tablespoons red wine vinegar
- 1½ tablespoons sugar
- 1 tablespoon canola or corn oil
- ⅜ teaspoon salt
- ¼ teaspoon pepper

1. In a medium bowl, gently toss together the salad ingredients.

2. In a small bowl, whisk together the dressing ingredients until the sugar is dissolved. Pour over the salad, tossing to coat. Serve immediately for peak flavor and texture.

3. Refrigerate the remaining beans in separate airtight containers for up to two days or freeze in airtight freezer containers for up to one month.

SODIUM SMARTS: This recipe, a healthy remake of the salty favorite, three-bean salad, calls for three kinds of canned *no-salt-added* beans. Using the no-salt-added instead of regular canned beans saves you at least 300 to 400 mg of sodium per serving.

PER SERVING
Calories 110
Total Fat 2.5 g
Saturated Fat 0.0 g
Trans Fat 0.0 g
Polyunsaturated Fat 0.5 g
Monounsaturated Fat 1.5 g
Cholesterol 0 mg
Sodium 148 mg
Carbohydrates 18 g
Fiber 4 g
Sugars 6 g
Protein 5 g
Calcium 42 mg
Potassium 331 mg
Dietary Exchanges:
1 starch, 1 vegetable, ½ fat

Garlic-Dill Potato Salad

Vinaigrette replaces mayonnaise in this version of potato salad. Wait until serving time to add the dressing so you'll get the pungent vinegar kick.

SERVES 6
½ cup per serving

SALAD

- 8 cups water
- 4 or 5 small red potatoes (12 ounces total)
- ½ cup chopped red or yellow onion
- ½ medium rib of celery, finely chopped

DRESSING

- 2 to 3 tablespoons cider vinegar
- 2 tablespoons olive oil (extra virgin preferred)
- 1 teaspoon dried dillweed, crumbled
- 2 medium garlic cloves, minced
- ¼ teaspoon salt
- ⅛ teaspoon crushed red pepper flakes

1. In a large saucepan, bring the water to a boil over high heat. Add the potatoes. Return to a boil. Boil for 18 minutes, or until just tender when pierced with a fork. Drain well in a colander. Let cool to room temperature, about 1 hour. Transfer the potatoes to a cutting board. Chop the potatoes. Transfer to a medium bowl.

2. Stir in the onion and celery.

3. In a small bowl, whisk together the dressing ingredients. Pour over the potato salad, stirring gently to combine. Serve immediately for peak flavor and texture.

PER SERVING
Calories 93
Total Fat 4.5 g
Saturated Fat 0.5 g
Trans Fat 0.0 g
Polyunsaturated Fat 0.5 g
Monounsaturated Fat 3.5 g
Cholesterol 0 mg
Sodium 105 mg
Carbohydrates 12 g
Fiber 2 g
Sugars 1 g
Protein 1 g
Calcium 281 mg
Potassium 17 mg
Dietary Exchanges:
1 starch, 1 fat

Curried Tuna Salad with Almonds

Try scoops of this curried tuna salad as part of a salad plate, or wrap them in crisp Bibb lettuce leaves.

SERVES 6
⅔ cup per serving

- 2 4.5-ounce cans very low sodium albacore tuna, packed in water, rinsed, well drained, and flaked
- ⅓ cup light mayonnaise
- 2 tablespoons fat-free milk
- 2 teaspoons curry powder
- ½ teaspoon ground cumin
- 2 medium ribs of celery, finely chopped
- ½ cup slivered almonds, dry-roasted
- ⅓ cup raisins

1. In a medium bowl, stir together the tuna, mayonnaise, milk, curry powder, and cumin.

2. Gently stir in the celery, almonds, and raisins, keeping the mixture fluffy rather than packing it down.

SODIUM SMARTS: Now that very low sodium canned tuna (about 45 mg of sodium in 3 ounces, compared to about 315 mg in the regular variety) is widely available, you can easily take in all the healthful benefits tuna has to offer while leaving out unwanted sodium.

PER SERVING
Calories 162
Total Fat 8.5 g
Saturated Fat 0.5 g
Trans Fat 0.0 g
Polyunsaturated Fat 0.5 g
Monounsaturated Fat 3.5 g
Cholesterol 23 mg
Sodium 158 mg
Carbohydrates 11 g
Fiber 2 g
Sugars 6 g
Protein 14 g
Calcium 50 mg
Potassium 296 mg
Dietary Exchanges:
1 fruit, 2 lean meat, ½ fat

Coleslaw with Ginger and Celery Seeds

This salad complements a variety of Asian dishes as well as grilled burgers, steaks, chicken, and seafood. It's perfect for summer gatherings because it isn't mayonnaise based.

SERVES 8
½ cup per serving

SLAW

- 4 cups coleslaw mix (about 8 ounces)
- ½ cup matchstick-size carrot strips or 1 medium carrot, coarsely shredded
- ½ medium green bell pepper, diced

DRESSING

- 3 tablespoons plain rice wine vinegar or white vinegar
- 2 tablespoons firmly packed light brown sugar
- 1 tablespoon grated peeled gingerroot
- 2 teaspoons canola or corn oil
- ½ to 1 teaspoon celery seeds
- ⅛ teaspoon salt

1. In a large bowl, toss together the slaw ingredients.

2. In a small bowl, whisk together the dressing ingredients until the brown sugar is dissolved. Pour over the slaw, tossing to coat. Serve immediately for peak flavor.

SODIUM SMARTS: The low-sodium dressing in this coleslaw replaces light mayonnaise, not only making for an unusual, crisp, and refreshing coleslaw but also saving you about 120 mg of sodium for each tablespoon of light mayonnaise you replace.

PER SERVING

Calories 38
Total Fat 1.5 g
Saturated Fat 0.0 g
Trans Fat 0.0 g
Polyunsaturated Fat 0.5 g
Monounsaturated Fat 1.0 g
Cholesterol 0 mg
Sodium 50 mg
Carbohydrates 7 g
Fiber 1 g
Sugars 5 g
Protein 1 g
Calcium 24 mg
Potassium 107 mg
Dietary Exchanges:
1 vegetable, ½ fat

Ranch-Style Dressing with Green Onions

Try this lower-sodium version of ever-popular ranch dressing on mixed salad greens, sliced tomatoes and cucumbers, or steamed vegetables, such as broccoli or carrots.

SERVES 8
2 tablespoons per serving

- **⅓ cup light mayonnaise**
- **¼ cup fat-free sour cream**
- **¼ cup fat-free milk**
- **1½ tablespoons cider vinegar**
- **2 medium garlic cloves, minced**
- **½ teaspoon onion powder**
- **½ teaspoon dry mustard**
- **½ teaspoon pepper (coarsely ground preferred)**
- **¼ teaspoon salt**
- **2 tablespoons finely chopped green onions**

1. For a dressing with a bit of texture, in a small bowl, whisk together all the ingredients except the green onions. Whisk in the green onions. For a smooth texture, process all the ingredients in a small food processor or blender until the desired consistency. Transfer the dressing to a jar with a tight-fitting lid. Refrigerate for at least 2 hours so the flavors blend.

2. Refrigerate leftover dressing in a covered jar for up to two weeks.

PER SERVING
Calories 47
Total Fat 3.5 g
Saturated Fat 0.5 g
Trans Fat 0.0 g
Polyunsaturated Fat 2.0 g
Monounsaturated Fat 1.0 g
Cholesterol 5 mg
Sodium 152 mg
Carbohydrates 3 g
Fiber 0 g
Sugars 1 g
Protein 1 g
Calcium 48 mg
Potassium 30 mg
Dietary Exchanges: 1 fat

Basil-Garlic Italian Dressing

While you process the ingredients for this dressing, watch as the fresh basil turns it an appealing bright green. The ingredients are so flavorful that you don't need to use any salt.

SERVES 8
2 tablespoons per serving

14 small pimiento-stuffed green olives, drained
½ cup dry white wine (regular or nonalcoholic)
¼ cup chopped fresh basil or 2 teaspoons dried basil, crumbled
¼ cup olive oil (extra virgin preferred)
¼ cup cider vinegar
1 teaspoon dry mustard
1 teaspoon snipped fresh rosemary or ⅛ teaspoon dried rosemary, crushed
2 medium garlic cloves
½ teaspoon sugar
¼ teaspoon crushed red pepper flakes

In a small food processor or a blender, process all the ingredients until smooth. Transfer to a jar with a tight-fitting lid. Refrigerate and use on the day you make the dressing if using fresh herbs or keep it for up to two weeks if using dried herbs.

SODIUM SMARTS: Two tablespoons of most bottled salad dressings are loaded with salt and contain hundreds of milligrams of sodium. Watch out for the low-fat or fat-free varieties, because they can contain even more added salt.

PER SERVING
Calories 83
Total Fat 8.0 g
Saturated Fat 1.0 g
Trans Fat 0.0 g
Polyunsaturated Fat 1.0 g
Monounsaturated Fat 6.0 g
Cholesterol 0 mg
Sodium 146 mg
Carbohydrates 1 g
Fiber 0 g
Sugars 0 g
Protein 0 g
Calcium 12 mg
Potassium 35 mg
Dietary Exchanges:
1½ fat

Thousand Island Dressing

Thousand Island dressing has stood the test of time and remains popular today. Try our lighter, lower-in-sodium version—it has just the right balance of creamy, sweet, and spicy!

SERVES 8
2 tablespoons per serving

- ¼ cup plus 2 tablespoons fat-free plain Greek yogurt
- 3 tablespoons light mayonnaise salad dressing or light mayonnaise
- 3 tablespoons no-salt-added ketchup
- 1½ tablespoons undrained sweet pickle relish (lowest sodium available)
- 1 tablespoon dehydrated minced onion
- 1 tablespoon chili sauce (lowest sodium available)
- White of 1 large hard-cooked egg, finely chopped, yolk discarded

1. In a small bowl, whisk together all the ingredients. Cover and refrigerate for at least 1 hour so the flavors blend.

2. Refrigerate leftover dressing in an airtight container for no more than two days.

SODIUM SMARTS: Ketchup can add about 170 mg of sodium per tablespoon to any dish. In this recipe, that could total as much as 510 mg, so be sure to use the no-salt-added or at least the low-sodium variety.

PER SERVING

Calories 34
Total Fat 1.5 g
Saturated Fat 1.0 g
Trans Fat 0.0 g
Polyunsaturated Fat 1.0 g
Monounsaturated Fat 0.5 g
Cholesterol 2 mg
Sodium 113 mg
Carbohydrates 4 g
Fiber 0 g
Sugars 4 g
Protein 2 g
Calcium 10 mg
Potassium 60 mg
Dietary Exchanges: Free

VEGETABLES AND FRUITS

Vegetables and fruits contain extremely low amounts of sodium (if any at all) and provide essential fiber, vitamins, and minerals. Sodium often comes into play, however, when these foods are processed. Whether salt is added during canning or in the form of sauces and seasonings, processing alters the natural flavor of these nutritious foods and the sodium content goes up. (Most frozen vegetables without sauces do not contain added salt.) Look at the chart on the following page to compare the sodium values of the fresh, canned, and no-salt-added canned and frozen varieties of some common vegetables.

TRY THESE LOWER-SODIUM VEGETABLE SIDE-DISH RECIPES:

- Creamy Corn with Onions (page 230)
- Scalloped Potato Casserole (page 231)
- Two-Potato Unfried French Fries (page 232)
- Green Bean Casserole (page 233)

SPOTLIGHT ON: Canned Green Beans

One of the most popular vegetables in America, canned green beans are also high in sodium. A half-cup of canned green beans contains, on average, about 350 mg of sodium—more than 20 percent of the daily recommended amount. By comparison, ½ cup of green beans in their raw, unprocessed state contains only about 5 mg of sodium. If you look for reduced-sodium canned green beans, you can save an average of 170 mg per serving. For further sodium savings, select no-salt-added canned green beans or fresh or frozen green beans.

SODIUM IN SELECTED VEGETABLES AND FRUITS

FOOD	SODIUM (MG)*
fresh fruits, such as apples, bananas, berries, and oranges	0
green beans, canned, ½ cup	295–400
green beans, canned, reduced-sodium, ½ cup	170–190
green beans, canned, no-salt-added, ½ cup	5–20
green beans, fresh or frozen, 4 oz	5
tomatoes, canned, ½ cup	160–310
tomatoes, canned, no-salt-added, ½ cup	10–50
tomato, fresh, 1 medium	5
dried beans, any variety, 1 oz	0
black beans, canned, ½ cup	350–565
black beans, canned, reduced-sodium, ½ cup	210–230
black beans, canned, no-salt-added, ½ cup	0–15
pinto beans, canned, ½ cup	220–475
pinto beans, canned, reduced-sodium, ½ cup	190
pinto beans, canned, no-salt-added, ½ cup	15
Creamy Corn with Onions (page 230), ½ cup	130
corn, creamed, frozen or canned, ½ cup	300–355
corn, canned, ½ cup	250–360
corn, canned, reduced-sodium, ½ cup	170–180
corn, fresh kernels, ½ cup	15
celery, fresh, 4 oz	90
carrots, fresh, 4 oz	80
beets, fresh, 4 oz	90
chard, fresh, 4 oz	240
spinach, fresh, 4 oz	90
french fries, frozen, 4 oz	305–460
Two-Potato Unfried French Fries (page 232), ½ cup	185
scalloped potato mix, 1 oz	385–620
Scalloped Potato Casserole (page 231), ½ cup	165

***Sodium values have been rounded to the nearest 5 mg.**

SODIUM-SAVING SOLUTIONS

- Look for no-salt-added or reduced-sodium canned vegetables; they can save you a *lot* of sodium.
- When shopping for canned or frozen vegetables, avoid buying those labeled "seasoned" or "flavored"; these will likely contain much more sodium than the unseasoned versions. Unseasoned, unsauced frozen vegetables are very nutritious because they are usually flash-frozen at the peak of their freshness. However, avoid frozen veggies that are prepared with seasonings or sauces because those can be loaded with salt. Be sure to read the nutrition facts panels for the sodium value. Remember, you have the control to put the flavor in, but you can't take out the sodium added in processing.
- Regular canned beans, such as black, pinto, and kidney, are also very high in sodium, so look for labels that say "no salt added" or "reduced sodium."
- Instead of reaching for the saltshaker, experiment with combinations of garlic, onion, and herbs such as parsley, dill, and tarragon to help flavor your veggies.
- Instead of dousing corn with salt, try brushing it with a combination of chopped basil, minced garlic, and a small amount of melted light tub margarine. This combination is so flavorful that you won't miss the salt.
- Add a pinch of sugar or a squeeze of fresh lemon juice to help bring out the vegetables' natural flavors.
- When soaking or cooking dried beans, don't add salt to the water. It may toughen the beans and prevent the water from being absorbed.
- Instant potatoes and potato mixes packaged with sauces or seasonings, such as for au gratin or scalloped potatoes, are high in sodium.
- If you can't find no-salt-added or reduced-sodium versions of canned beans and vegetables, pour the regular kind into a colander and rinse them to remove about 10 percent of the sodium.
- Try roasting vegetables to bring out their natural flavors.

Creamy Corn with Onions

Here's a scrumptious accompaniment to any entrée that's all about rich-tasting, creamy comfort, but that's lower in sodium and calories than many similar dishes.

SERVES 4
½ cup per serving

- Cooking spray
- ½ cup chopped onion
- 1 15.25-ounce can no-salt-added whole-kernel corn, drained
- ¼ cup fat-free milk
- 3 tablespoons whipped light tub cream cheese (about 1½ ounces)
- ¼ teaspoon pepper
- ⅛ teaspoon salt
- 1 medium green onion, finely chopped (optional)

1. Lightly spray a medium saucepan with cooking spray. Cook the onion over medium heat for 3 minutes, stirring frequently.

2. Stir in the corn, milk, and cream cheese. Bring just to a boil, still over medium heat. Reduce the heat and simmer, covered, for 10 minutes, or until the mixture has thickened slightly and the onion is very soft. Remove from the heat.

3. Let stand, uncovered, for at least 5 minutes so the mixture thickens and the rich cream cheese flavor intensifies. Stir in the pepper and salt. Sprinkle with the green onion.

PER SERVING
Calories 98
Total Fat 1.5 g
Saturated Fat 1.0 g
Trans Fat 0.0 g
Polyunsaturated Fat 0.5 g
Monounsaturated Fat 0.5 g
Cholesterol 4 mg
Sodium 128 mg
Carbohydrates 20 g
Fiber 2 g
Sugars 5 g
Protein 3 g
Calcium 39 mg
Potassium 251 mg
Dietary Exchanges:
1½ starch

Scalloped Potato C

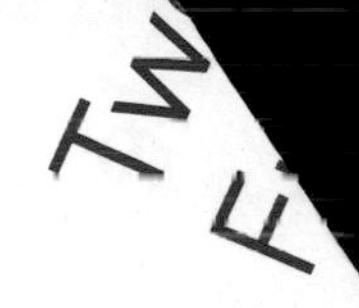

Dress up simple roasts, such as Espresso Eye
with this colorful root-veggie side dish.

SERVES 6
½ cup per serving

- Cooking spray
- 12 ounces golden potatoes (about 2 medium), very thinly sliced crosswise
- 1 small fennel bulb, thinly sliced (about 1 cup)
- ½ medium red bell pepper, cut lengthwise into thin strips, then cut crosswise into 2-inch pieces
- ½ cup chopped onion
- ½ cup matchstick-size carrot strips
- ½ teaspoon dried thyme, crumbled
- 2 tablespoons all-purpose flour
- ½ cup fat-free milk
- 2 tablespoons light tub margarine
- ½ teaspoon pepper
- ¼ teaspoon ground nutmeg
- ¼ teaspoon salt

1. Preheat the oven to 350°F. Lightly
9-inch square glass baking dish and a piece
aluminum foil large enough to cover the dish with cooking spray. Set the foil aside.

2. Arrange half the potato slices in the dish. Top, in order, with all the fennel, bell pepper, onion, and carrot. Sprinkle with the thyme. Top with the remaining potato slices.

3. Put the flour in a small bowl. Pour in the milk, whisking to dissolve. Pour over the potato mixture.

4. Dot the top with the margarine, divided into 12 pieces, each about ½ teaspoon. Sprinkle the pepper and nutmeg over all. Cover the baking dish with the foil with the sprayed side down.

5. Bake for 40 minutes. Remove the foil. Bake for 25 minutes, or until the potatoes are very tender. Remove from the oven.

6. Sprinkle the casserole with the salt. Let stand for 10 minutes so the flavors blend and the liquid is absorbed.

PER SERVING

Calories 99	Carbohydrates 19 g
Total Fat 2.0 g	Fiber 3 g
Saturated Fat 0.0 g	Sugars 3 g
Trans Fat 0.0 g	Protein 3 g
Polyunsaturated Fat 0.5 g	Calcium 514 mg
Monounsaturated Fat 1.0 g	Potassium 60 mg
Cholesterol 0 mg	Dietary Exchanges:
Sodium 167 mg	1 starch, 1 vegetable

o-Potato Unfried rench Fries

Seasoned generously with fresh herbs, onion powder, garlic powder, and pepper, plus just a small amount of salt, these rough-cut, colorful fries are an excellent replacement for salt-laden fast-food french fries.

SERVES 4
½ cup per serving

- Cooking spray
- 1 large unpeeled red potato (about 8 ounces), cut lengthwise into ½-inch-wide strips
- 1 medium sweet potato (about 8 ounces), peeled, cut lengthwise into ½-inch-wide strips
- 1 tablespoon canola or corn oil
- 1 teaspoon snipped fresh rosemary or ¼ teaspoon dried rosemary, crushed
- ¾ teaspoon snipped fresh thyme or ¼ teaspoon dried thyme, crumbled
- ½ teaspoon onion powder
- ¼ teaspoon garlic powder
- ¼ teaspoon pepper
- ¼ teaspoon salt

1. Preheat the oven to 425°F. Lightly spray a large baking sheet with cooking spray.

2. In a large bowl, gently stir together all the ingredients except the salt. Spread the potatoes in a single layer on the baking sheet.

3. Roast for 15 minutes. Using a wide spatula, turn the potatoes over (it's fine if you don't turn every piece). Roast for 10 minutes, or until the potatoes are tender and browned. Remove from the oven. Leaving the potatoes on the baking sheet, sprinkle with the salt. Serve immediately for peak flavor and texture.

PER SERVING
Calories 122
Total Fat 3.5 g
Saturated Fat 0.5 g
Trans Fat 0.0 g
Polyunsaturated Fat 1.0 g
Monounsaturated Fat 2.0 g
Cholesterol 0 mg
Sodium 187 mg
Carbohydrates 21 g
Fiber 3 g
Sugars 3 g
Protein 2 g
Calcium 27 mg
Potassium 458 mg
Dietary Exchanges:
1½ starch, ½ fat

Green Bean Casserole

By replacing canned cream of mushroom soup with your own easy, herb-infused white sauce and using sautéed onion instead of canned fried onion rings on top, you can keep the sodium and fat in check in this classic side dish.

SERVES 8
½ cup per serving

- 1 tablespoon olive oil
- 2 tablespoons all-purpose flour
- 2 teaspoons fresh thyme or 1 teaspoon dried Italian seasoning, crumbled
- ¼ teaspoon salt
- ¼ teaspoon pepper
- 1 cup fat-free milk
- ½ cup finely chopped onion
- 4 ounces button mushrooms, sliced
- 1 medium garlic clove, minced
- 16 ounces frozen French-cut green beans, thawed
- ½ cup plain whole-wheat panko

1. Preheat the oven to 375°F.

2. In a medium saucepan, heat the oil over medium heat, swirling to coat the bottom. Whisk in the flour, thyme, salt, and pepper. Cook for 1 minute, whisking constantly. Gradually whisk in the milk. Cook for 4 to 5 minutes, or until thickened and bubbly, whisking constantly. Set the white sauce aside.

3. In a large nonstick skillet, cook the onion over medium heat for 4 minutes, or until soft, stirring frequently. Transfer ¼ cup of the onion to a small plate. Set aside.

4. Stir the mushrooms and garlic into the onion remaining in the skillet. Cook for 4 to 5 minutes, or until the mushrooms are soft, stirring occasionally. Stir the mushroom mixture and beans into the white sauce. Transfer to a 1½-quart glass casserole dish. Sprinkle the panko and reserved ¼ cup onion over the top.

5. Bake for 25 to 30 minutes, or until the sauce is bubbly and the panko is golden.

PER SERVING
Calories 80
Total Fat 2.0 g
Saturated Fat 0.5 g
Trans Fat 0.0 g
Polyunsaturated Fat 0.5 g
Monounsaturated Fat 1.0 g
Cholesterol 1 mg
Sodium 94 mg
Carbohydrates 12 g
Fiber 2 g
Sugars 4 g
Protein 4 g
Calcium 68 mg
Potassium 215 mg
Dietary Exchanges:
½ starch, 1 vegetable, ½ fat

BREAKFAST FOODS

Cereal is a fast and easy breakfast choice and can have health benefits, especially if you select a whole-grain variety. However, many cereals also contain a lot of sodium, so be sure to compare nutrition facts panels. Other popular breakfast foods that can be high in sodium are baked goods such as muffins or croissants and bread products such as English muffins or bagels. (See page 131 for more information on breads.) The sodium values in the chart on the following page will show you how easily sodium can add up at the first meal of the day.

TRY THESE LOWER-SODIUM BREAKFAST RECIPES:

- Apricot and Orange Muffins (page 237)
- Pancakes with Blueberry-Vanilla Sauce (page 238)
- Easy and Heart-y Oatmeal Mix (page 240)
- Open-Face Breakfast Sandwiches (page 241)

SPOTLIGHT ON: Cereals If you eat fortified whole-grain cereal with milk, you get not only the grains but also calcium, so what's the health concern? Just because a cereal doesn't taste salty doesn't mean it's not jam-packed with sodium; in fact, packaged ready-to-eat cereals can contain a surprising amount. With so many choices on the shelves, take some time to compare labels and find lower-sodium products.

SODIUM IN SELECTED BREAKFAST FOODS

FOOD	SODIUM (MG)*
bran flakes, plain, 1 oz	190–230
raisin bran, sweetened, 1 oz	120
cornflakes, 1 oz	200–270
puffed rice, 1 oz	0
granola, 1 oz	0–105
shredded wheat, 1 oz	0
pancake mix, ¼ cup; 2 pancakes and 2 tbsp pancake syrup	330–455
Pancakes with Blueberry-Vanilla Sauce (page 238), 2 pancakes, ⅓ cup sauce, and 2 tbsp yogurt	305
instant oatmeal, maple and brown sugar flavor, single-serving packet	100–260
Easy and Heart-y Oatmeal Mix (page 240), 1 cup	40
fruit muffin, 4 oz	350–420
Apricot and Orange Muffins (page 237), 1 muffin	90
coffeecake, 2 oz	160–240
fruit turnover, 2 oz	250–260
waffle, frozen	165–310
egg substitute, ¼ cup, equal to 1 large egg	120–125
egg, whole, large	70
doughnut, cake type, plain, 3¼-inch	280–340
breakfast sandwich, frozen	480–800
Open-Face Breakfast Sandwiches (page 241), 1 sandwich	295

***Sodium values have been rounded to the nearest 5 mg.**

SODIUM-SAVING SOLUTIONS

- When buying cereals, compare nutrition facts panels and choose ones with lower amounts of sodium. Also, choose cereals that list whole grains, such as whole wheat or whole oats, as the first ingredient. Cereals can be a good source of fiber, so look for those that contain at least 3 grams of fiber per serving; better yet, a cereal with 5 grams or more is considered a high-fiber source.
- Don't be lulled by the front-of-package labeling into thinking that a cereal is low in sodium because the label says it is "healthy." Terms such as "fat-free," "low-fat," or "organic" do not mean low in salt as well.
- Some cereals contain no sodium. Look for plain cream of wheat (not instant), grits, quick or old-fashioned oatmeal (not instant), puffed rice, puffed wheat, and most shredded wheat cereals.
- Although egg substitutes are much lower in cholesterol than eggs, they contain nearly twice as much sodium; choose the one that best meets your overall needs.
- Bacon is high in sodium as well as saturated fat, so consider eating this only once in a while. Instead, try low-fat breakfast sausages or turkey bacon, each of which will reduce your intake of unhealthy fats and save from 55 to 200 mg of sodium per serving.
- Breakfast dishes that are made from a mix, such as pancakes, waffles, or muffins, will contain sodium, so be sure to compare nutrition facts panels and choose from the products with the lowest amounts. To really cut back, make your own mixes. (See our muffin and pancake recipes on pages 237 and 238.)
- Pancake syrups contain sodium, so look for the lowest sodium available, choose 100 percent pure maple syrup or honey, or try topping your waffles or pancakes with fresh fruit, fat-free yogurt, and a dash of cinnamon instead. If you opt for maple syrup or honey, use them sparingly as they can quickly add calories.
- For an easy low-sodium breakfast to kick off your day, mix your choice of fresh fruit into fat-free plain or Greek-style yogurt.

Apricot and Orange Muffins

Dried apricot bits add bursts of flavor to these slightly sweet muffins, and the toasted wheat germ adds crunch and a delicious nutty taste.

SERVES 8
1 muffin or 3 mini muffins per serving

- Cooking spray
- ¾ cup whole-wheat flour
- ¾ cup all-purpose flour
- ½ cup firmly packed light brown sugar
- ⅓ cup toasted wheat germ and 2 tablespoons toasted wheat germ, divided use
- 1½ teaspoons baking powder
- 1 teaspoon ground cinnamon
- ⅓ cup chopped dried apricots
- ¾ cup fresh orange juice
- 1 large egg
- 3 tablespoons unsweetened applesauce
- 1½ tablespoons canola or corn oil
- ½ teaspoon vanilla extract

1. Preheat the oven to 375°F. Lightly spray 8 cups of a standard 12-cup muffin pan or two 12-cup mini muffin pans with cooking spray.

2. In a medium bowl, stir together the flours, brown sugar, ⅓ cup wheat germ, baking powder, and cinnamon. Stir in the apricots.

3. In a small bowl, whisk together the remaining ingredients except the remaining 2 tablespoons wheat germ. Pour into the flour mixture, stirring until the batter is just moistened but no flour is visible. Don't overmix; the batter should be slightly lumpy.

4. Spoon about ⅓ cup batter into each of the 8 standard muffin cups or 1 heaping tablespoon batter into each of the 24 mini muffin cups. Sprinkle the remaining wheat germ over the batter.

5. Bake the muffins for 22 to 24 minutes or the mini muffins for 12 to 14 minutes, or until a wooden toothpick inserted in the center of a muffin or mini muffin comes out clean. Transfer the pan(s) to a cooling rack and let cool completely, at least 30 minutes.

PER SERVING
Calories 218
Total Fat 4.5 g
Saturated Fat 0.5 g
Trans Fat 0.0 g
Polyunsaturated Fat 1.5 g
Monounsaturated Fat 2.0 g
Cholesterol 23 mg
Sodium 89 mg
Carbohydrates 41 g
Fiber 3 g
Sugars 20 g
Protein 6 g
Calcium 78 mg
Potassium 258 mg
Dietary Exchanges:
2½ other carbohydrate, 1 fat

Pancakes with Blueberry-Vanilla Sauce

You can prepare the batter in advance, making it easy to put a delicious hot breakfast on the table in short order.

SERVES 4
2 pancakes, ⅓ cup sauce, and 2 tablespoons yogurt per serving

SAUCE

- 2 teaspoons cornstarch
- ⅓ cup water
- 1 cup blueberries
- 1½ tablespoons sugar
- 1½ teaspoons vanilla extract

PANCAKES

- 1 cup white whole-wheat flour
- 1½ tablespoons sugar
- 2 teaspoons baking powder
- 1 cup low-fat buttermilk
- 2 large egg whites
- 1 tablespoon grated lemon zest
- 1 tablespoon plus 1 teaspoon canola or corn oil
- 1 teaspoon vanilla extract

- ½ cup fat-free plain Greek yogurt

1. If your griddle isn't large enough to cook 8 pancakes at once, preheat the oven to 200°F. Place a cooling rack on a baking sheet. Set aside.

2. Put the cornstarch in a medium saucepan. Add the water, stirring to dissolve. Stir in the blueberries and 1½ tablespoons sugar. Bring to a boil over medium-high heat. Boil for 1 minute. Remove from the heat.

3. Stir in 1½ teaspoons vanilla. Cover to keep warm. Set the sauce aside.

4. In a medium bowl, stir together the flour, remaining 1½ tablespoons sugar, and the baking powder.

5. In a small bowl, whisk together the buttermilk, egg whites, lemon zest, oil, and remaining 1 teaspoon vanilla. Stir into the flour mixture just until combined but no flour is visible. Don't overmix; the batter should be slightly lumpy.

6. Heat a nonstick griddle over medium heat. Test the temperature by sprinkling a few drops of water on the griddle. If the water evaporates quickly, the griddle is ready. Pour ¼ cup batter for each pancake onto the griddle. Cook for 2 minutes, or until bubbles appear all over the surface and the bottoms are golden brown. Turn the pancakes over. Cook for 1 to 2 minutes, or until cooked through and golden brown on the bottoms. If you have more batter to use, place the pancakes in a single layer on the cooling rack, leaving some space between them. Transfer to the oven to keep warm. Repeat with the remaining batter (you should have a total of 8 pancakes).

7. Transfer the pancakes to plates. Spoon the blueberry sauce over the pancakes. Top each serving with 2 tablespoons yogurt.

8. You can prepare the pancake batter up to two days in advance, refrigerate it in an airtight container, cook just the amount you need, and save the rest. The sauce, however, has the best texture and flavor on the day you make it. If you use the pancake batter for several breakfasts, you can make part of the sauce for each meal or substitute pure maple syrup (pancake syrups contain sodium).

PER SERVING

Calories 263	Carbohydrates 42 g
Total Fat 6.0 g	Fiber 4 g
Saturated Fat 1.0 g	Sugars 18 g
Trans Fat 0.0 g	Protein 11 g
Polyunsaturated Fat 1.5 g	Calcium 334 mg
Monounsaturated Fat 3.0 g	Potassium 226 mg
Cholesterol 3 mg	Dietary Exchanges:
Sodium 304 mg	2 starch, 1 fruit, 1 fat

Easy and Heart-y Oatmeal Mix

Make yourself a filling breakfast without missing a beat. For a single serving of this oatmeal, just add water to a small amount of the mix, then microwave the oatmeal or cook it on the stovetop. The dry mix stores well (up to one month in an airtight container in a cool, dry place), so keep some on hand.

MAKES 6 CUPS DRY MIX
enough for nine 1-cup servings prepared

- **3½ cups uncooked quick-cooking oatmeal**
- **1 cup sweetened dried cranberries, dried cherries, raisins, dried apples, or any combination**
- **¾ cup fat-free dry milk**
- **½ cup firmly packed light brown sugar**
- **½ cup chopped pecans**
- **1½ tablespoons ground cinnamon**
- **¼ teaspoon ground allspice**

1. In a large bowl, stir together all the ingredients, breaking up any clumps of dried fruit pieces and brown sugar.

2. To microwave a single serving of the oatmeal, in a microwaveable bowl with at least a 3-cup capacity (the oatmeal needs room to expand), stir together ⅔ cup oatmeal mix and ¾ to 1 cup water, depending on whether you prefer thicker or thinner oatmeal. Microwave on 100 percent power (high) for 2 to 2½ minutes, or until the oatmeal is bubbly and starting to thicken. Remove from the microwave. Let cool for 1 minute, stirring once halfway through.

3. To cook the oatmeal on the stovetop, in a small saucepan, bring ¾ to 1 cup water to a boil over high heat. Slowly stir in ⅔ cup of the mix. Reduce the heat to medium and cook for 1 minute, stirring constantly. Remove from the heat. Let stand, covered, for 1 minute, or until the oatmeal reaches the desired consistency.

PER SERVING

Calories 278	Carbohydrates 49 g
Total Fat 6.5 g	Fiber 5 g
Saturated Fat 0.5 g	Sugars 26 g
Trans Fat 0.0 g	Protein 8 g
Polyunsaturated Fat 2.0 g	Calcium 127 mg
Monounsaturated Fat 3.0 g	Potassium 265 mg
Cholesterol 0 mg	Dietary Exchanges:
Sodium 39 mg	2 starch, 1 fruit, 1 fat

Open-Face Breakfast Sandwiches

By making breakfast sandwiches at home (instead of buying them at a drive-through), and pairing them with fresh fruit, you can enjoy a delicious meal that gets your day off to a quick start.

SERVES 4
1 sandwich per serving

- 1 teaspoon canola or corn oil
- 1 medium green bell pepper, chopped
- 4 large eggs
- ¼ cup fat-free milk
- ½ teaspoon pepper
- ½ cup grape tomatoes, quartered
- 2 medium green onions, finely chopped
- ⅛ teaspoon salt
- 4 slices light whole-grain bread (lowest sodium available), lightly toasted
- ¼ cup shredded low-fat sharp Cheddar cheese

1. In a medium nonstick skillet, heat the oil over medium heat, swirling to coat the bottom. Cook the bell pepper for 3 minutes, or until beginning to soften, stirring frequently.

2. Meanwhile, in a medium bowl, whisk together the eggs, milk, and pepper. Pour over the bell pepper. Reduce the heat to medium low. Cook for 1½ minutes, or until the mixture is almost set, stirring occasionally. Gently stir in the tomatoes and green onions. Remove the skillet from the heat. Sprinkle the salt over the egg mixture.

3. Put the toast slices on plates. Spoon the egg mixture onto the toast. Sprinkle with the Cheddar.

PER SERVING
Calories 164
Total Fat 7.0 g
Saturated Fat 2.0 g
Trans Fat 0.0 g
Polyunsaturated Fat 1.5 g
Monounsaturated Fat 3.0 g
Cholesterol 188 mg
Sodium 296 mg
Carbohydrates 14 g
Fiber 2 g
Sugars 4 g
Protein 11 g
Calcium 302 mg
Potassium 102 mg
Dietary Exchanges:
1 starch, 1 lean meat, ½ fat

BEVERAGES

Most people probably think of sugar as the dietary villain in sweetened beverages; however, certain drinks can really add to your sodium intake as well. Most soft drinks contain added sodium because salt helps mask the metallic or chemical aftertastes these products can have. Because almost no beverages taste salty, you are not likely to think of the sodium they contain. If your choices are relatively high in sodium and you drink them frequently, you can easily put your sodium intake way over the top. Regardless of whether you eat it or drink it, the sodium adds up. Check the chart that follows to see how your beverages of choice contribute to your daily sodium intake.

SPOTLIGHT ON: Tomato Juice Drinking vegetable or fruit juice seems like a sensible way to get vitamins and minerals in your daily diet, but it's also an easy way to consume way too much sodium. An 8-ounce serving of regular tomato juice can have about 700 mg of sodium—about half the daily recommended amount! By switching to a low-sodium version, you'll still get your nutrients *and* you'll save about 615 mg of sodium.

SODIUM IN SELECTED BEVERAGES

BEVERAGE (8 OZ)	SODIUM (MG)*
tomato juice	655–750
tomato juice, low-sodium	25–140
mixed-vegetable juice	360–620
mixed-vegetable juice, low-sodium	140–170
coconut water	250
sports drink	55–100
energy drink	30–205
club soda	45–60

BEVERAGE (8 OZ)	SODIUM (MG)*
seltzer	0
regular cola	5–50
diet cola	25–30
iced green tea	0–30
milk, fat-free	105
wine	10
beer	5
Bloody Mary mix	1,120–1,175

*Sodium values have been rounded to the nearest 5 mg.

SODIUM-SAVING SOLUTIONS

- Opt to drink tap or bottled water whenever possible in place of higher-sodium beverages. If you don't like the taste, flavor your glass of water with a squeeze or two of fresh lime, lemon, orange, or cucumber; several mint leaves; or a splash of unsweetened cranberry juice concentrate or unsweetened iced tea.
- Be aware that tap water contains sodium, with the levels varying widely from one location to another. In some areas, the water is softened by adding even more sodium. Check the sodium content in your local water supply through your town's utility department. Unfortunately, you can't rely on filtered water pitchers or filters on your faucet or fridge to help—they don't remove the sodium in the water.
- When buying bottled drinks, such as iced teas or juices, compare nutrition facts panels and choose the drinks with the lowest sodium.
- When a recipe calls for wine, be sure to use a table wine. Cooking wine, which often is located with vinegars, contains added salt and is very high in sodium. The same holds true for cooking sherry; use regular sherry to avoid unnecessary sodium.
- Love your favorite coffee shop's specialty drinks? If you've made it a habit to stop in every day before work for a latte or a mocha, for example, you may be adding hundreds of milligrams of sodium to your diet. Look online to get the nutrition information for your favorites.

DESSERTS AND BAKING PRODUCTS

As perhaps you assumed about beverages, you might also think that sugar—not salt—is the nutrient to be concerned about in sweets. After all, desserts don't typically taste salty, so how can sodium be an issue? A food doesn't have to taste salty to be a source of sodium. In fact, salt often is added to enhance the sweetness of desserts. Additionally, two of the biggest sodium culprits in many baked goods are baking soda and baking powder, both used as leavening agents. In the chart on the following page, you'll see where the sodium lurks in popular sweets.

TRY THESE LOWER-SODIUM DESSERT RECIPES:

- Oatmeal Piecrust (page 247)
- Luscious Lemon Sponge Puddings (page 248)
- Carrot Cake with Cream Cheese Frosting (page 250)
- Oatmeal-Raisin Drop Cookies (page 252)

SPOTLIGHT ON: Cake Mixes So convenient, so easy, and so many flavors to choose from, but did you know that cake mixes also have plenty of sodium? On average, a serving of cake from a mix has about 300 mg of sodium, plus another 50 to 95 mg or so for the canned frosting (2 tablespoons). Assuming that you stick with the serving size given in the nutrition facts panel, one slice of frosted cake could cost you about 25 percent—or more—of the total daily sodium recommendation.

SODIUM IN SELECTED DESSERTS AND BAKING PRODUCTS

FOOD	SODIUM (MG)*
piecrust (1/8 of a pie)	90–145
Oatmeal Piecrust (page 247), 1/8 of a pie	60
graham cracker crust, 1/8 of a pie	85–170
puff pastry shell	115–230
cake mix, 1/12 of a cake	280–355
frosting, canned, 2 tbsp	50–95
Carrot Cake with Cream Cheese Frosting (page 250), 1/16 of a cake	95
baking soda, 1 tsp	1,260
baking powder, 1 tsp	400
angel food cake, 1/12 of a cake	290–475
apple pie, 1/8 of a pie	140–300
bread pudding, 4 oz	125–210
instant pudding mix, sugar-free, prepared, 1/2 cup	225–415
Luscious Lemon Sponge Puddings (page 248), 1 pudding	90
Oatmeal-Raisin Drop Cookies (page 252), 2 cookies	80

***Sodium values have been rounded to the nearest 5 mg.**

SODIUM-SAVING SOLUTIONS

- It is best to limit your consumption of commercial baked goods since they often are loaded not only with sodium but also with saturated and trans fats and sugars that contribute no nutrients or measurable health value. Baked goods from a bakery or the bakery department of a grocery store may not provide nutrition facts labels, so you have no way of knowing the nutritional values of these foods. Enjoy them as special treats rather than part of your regular meal plan.
- Made-from-scratch angel food cakes use egg whites rather than baking powder and baking soda, which are sodium-rich leavening agents. Macaroons don't need leavening, so they, too, are good choices for sweet treats. Store-bought cakes and cookies, however, not only may use baking powder and baking soda but also may contain sodium from added salt or sodium preservatives.
- Baking soda and baking powder, frequently found in baked goods, are very high in sodium (per teaspoon, baking soda has about 1,260 mg of sodium and baking powder has about 400 mg). Sodium-free baking soda and sodium-free baking powder are available, but often only online or in health-food stores. If you choose to substitute sodium-free baking soda for the regular variety, be sure to double the amount called for in the recipe.
- The main source of sodium in pie usually is the crust. If the filling, not the crust, of a store-bought pie is the part you really enjoy, try scooping it out and serving it in a parfait dish. A better option is to prepare your own crust (see page 247) or make your favorite pie in another way. For example, if apple pie is your weakness, bake a healthy homemade apple crisp/crumble instead and save big on sodium.
- Most desserts that are prepared from mixes, such as baked goods and instant puddings, are loaded with sodium, so eat them occasionally or make your own from scratch.

Oatmeal Piecrust

If you like oatmeal cookies, you'll love this chewy piecrust made with quick-cooking oatmeal, whole-wheat flour, and almond meal (also known as almond flour). Bake as directed and fill with your favorite fruit, homemade pie filling or pudding (the mixes contain too much sodium), or fat-free frozen yogurt or ice cream.

SERVES 8
⅛ crust per serving

- Cooking spray
- 1 cup uncooked quick-cooking oatmeal
- ¼ cup whole-wheat flour
- ¼ cup almond meal, or almond flour, or finely ground almonds with skin
- 3 tablespoons firmly packed light brown sugar
- ½ teaspoon ground cinnamon
- ⅛ teaspoon salt
- 2 tablespoons trans-fat-free stick margarine, melted
- 3 tablespoons fresh orange juice

1. Preheat the oven to 400°F. Lightly spray a 9-inch pie pan with cooking spray. Set aside.

2. In a medium bowl, using a fork, stir together the oatmeal, whole-wheat flour, almond meal, brown sugar, cinnamon, and salt. Drizzle with the margarine. Work it into the oat mixture until well combined.

3. Still using the fork, stir in the orange juice, 1 tablespoon at a time, until the mixture is slightly crumbly. Transfer to the pie pan.

4. Lay over the dough a piece of plastic wrap or wax paper large enough to cover the pan; this is to keep the dough from sticking to your hands. Press the dough over the bottom and about three-fourths of the way up the side of the pan. Discard the plastic wrap or wax paper.

5. Bake the crust for 13 to 15 minutes, or until golden brown. Transfer the pan to a cooling rack and let the crust cool completely, about 1 hour, before filling.

PER SERVING

Calories 116
Total Fat 5.0 g
Saturated Fat 1.0 g
Trans Fat 0.0 g
Polyunsaturated Fat 2.0 g
Monounsaturated Fat 2.0 g
Cholesterol 0 mg
Sodium 62 mg
Carbohydrates 16 g
Fiber 2 g
Sugars 6 g
Protein 3 g
Calcium 21 mg
Potassium 89 mg
Dietary Exchanges: 1 starch, 1 fat

Luscious Lemon Sponge Puddings

The batter for this light and refreshing dessert separates nicely into two layers as it bakes, giving you an airy sponge cake on top and a tangy lemon pudding below. The puddings are baked in individual custard cups, so your portion control will be under control!

SERVES 5
1 pudding per serving

- Cooking spray
- ½ cup plus 2 tablespoons sugar
- 1 tablespoon trans-fat-free stick margarine
- 1 large egg
- 2 teaspoons grated lemon zest
- 3 tablespoons all-purpose flour
- 1 cup fat-free milk
- ¼ cup fresh lemon juice
- ½ teaspoon vanilla extract
- 3 large egg whites
- ⅛ teaspoon cream of tartar
- 1¼ cups sliced hulled strawberries
- 1 teaspoon confectioners' sugar

1. Preheat the oven to 350°F. Lightly spray five 6-ounce glass or ceramic custard cups or ramekins with cooking spray. Set aside.

2. In a medium mixing bowl, using an electric mixer on medium speed, beat the sugar and margarine for 30 seconds, or until combined.

3. Add the egg and lemon zest. Beat for 1 to 1½ minutes, or until smooth.

4. Add the flour. Beat for 20 seconds, or until combined.

5. Add the milk, lemon juice, and vanilla. Beat for 1 minute, or until blended. Set aside. Wash and dry the beaters.

6. In a small mixing bowl, using an electric mixer on medium-low speed, beat the egg whites until foamy. Add the cream of tartar. Increase the speed to medium high and continue beating until the mixture forms stiff but not dry peaks (the peaks don't fall when the beaters are lifted). Don't overbeat. Gently fold the egg whites into the batter until completely incorporated (no bits of whites are visible).

7. Ladle the mixture into the custard cups. Arrange the cups in a 13 x 9 x 2-inch baking pan. The cups shouldn't touch each other or the sides of the pan. Carefully pour in enough hot water to come at least halfway up the sides of the cups. (A little higher than halfway is acceptable, but not a little lower.)

8. Bake for 30 minutes, or until the puddings are golden and the centers barely jiggle when the cups are gently shaken. Remove the cups from the pan and place on a cooling rack. Let cool for 20 to 30 minutes. Serve warm or cover each pudding with plastic wrap and refrigerate for up to 24 hours (for peak flavor and texture, serve within 24 hours of preparation). Whether the puddings are warm or chilled, top with the strawberries and sprinkle with the confectioners' sugar just before serving.

SODIUM SMARTS: This recipe will indulge your craving for something sweet without subjecting you to the high sodium levels in instant pudding. One serving of this recipe has about 90 mg of sodium, but the same amount of instant lemon pudding has hundreds more.

PER SERVING

Calories 196
Total Fat 3.5 g
Saturated Fat 1.0 g
Trans Fat 0.0 g
Polyunsaturated Fat 1.0 g
Monounsaturated Fat 1.0 g
Cholesterol 38 mg
Sodium 88 mg
Carbohydrates 36 g
Fiber 1 g
Sugars 31 g
Protein 6 g
Calcium 76 mg
Potassium 218 mg
Dietary Exchanges:
2½ other carbohydrate, ½ fat

Carrot Cake with Cream Cheese Frosting

Cakes tend to be very high in sodium and unhealthy fats, so try our version of the ever-popular carrot cake for a decadent treat with only a fraction of the sodium traditionally found in cake mixes. If you prefer an unfrosted version, just dust the cake with 2 tablespoons of confectioners' sugar.

SERVES 16
2 x 3-inch piece per serving

- Cooking spray
- 2 tablespoons all-purpose flour

CAKE

- 4 large egg whites
- ½ cup sugar
- ½ cup firmly packed light brown sugar
- ½ cup unsweetened applesauce
- ½ cup fat-free milk
- 1 tablespoon canola or corn oil
- 1½ teaspoons vanilla extract
- 1¼ cups whole-wheat flour
- 1¼ cups all-purpose flour
- 1 tablespoon ground cinnamon
- 2 teaspoons baking powder
- ¼ teaspoon ground allspice
- 1½ cups grated carrots

CONTINUED

1. Preheat the oven to 350°F. Lightly spray a 13 x 9 x 2-inch baking pan with cooking spray. Sprinkle 2 tablespoons flour in the pan, shaking so the flour adheres to the sides and bottom. Shake out any excess flour.

2. In a medium mixing bowl, using an electric mixer on medium speed, beat the egg whites, sugars, applesauce, ½ cup milk, the oil, and 1½ teaspoons vanilla for 1 minute, or until combined.

3. In a medium bowl, stir together the whole-wheat flour, remaining 1¼ cups all-purpose flour, cinnamon, baking powder, and allspice. Gradually add the flour mixture to the egg white mixture while beating on medium speed for about 1 minute, or until blended.

4. Stir in the carrots, pineapple with liquid, and raisins. Pour into the pan, lightly smoothing the top.

5. Bake for 35 to 40 minutes, or until a wooden toothpick inserted in the center comes out clean. Transfer to a cooling rack and let cool for at least 1½ hours before frosting.

6. In a medium mixing bowl, using an electric mixer on medium speed, beat together the frosting ingredients except the pecans for 1 minute, or until smooth. Spread on the cooled cake. Sprinkle with the pecans. Serve the same day for peak flavor and texture.

7. Cover any leftovers and refrigerate for up to three days.

1 8-ounce can crushed pineapple in its own juice, undrained

½ cup raisins

FROSTING

2 cups unsifted confectioners' sugar

2 ounces low-fat brick-type cream cheese, softened (don't use fat free)

2 teaspoons fat-free milk

½ teaspoon vanilla extract

¼ cup finely chopped pecans or walnuts (dry-roasted preferred)

PER SERVING

WITH CREAM CHEESE FROSTING

Calories 248	Carbohydrates 53 g
Total Fat 3.0 g	Fiber 2 g
Saturated Fat 0.5 g	Sugars 35 g
Trans Fat 0.0 g	Protein 4 g
Polyunsaturated Fat 1.0 g	Calcium 71 mg
Monounsaturated Fat 1.5 g	Potassium 195 mg
Cholesterol 2 mg	Dietary Exchanges:
Sodium 95 mg	3½ other carbohydrate, ½ fat

WITH 2 TABLESPOONS CONFECTIONERS' SUGAR

Calories 174	Carbohydrates 38 g
Total Fat 1.5 g	Fiber 2 g
Saturated Fat 0.0 g	Sugars 21 g
Trans Fat 0.0 g	Protein 4 g
Polyunsaturated Fat 0.5 g	Calcium 64 mg
Monounsaturated Fat 0.5 g	Potassium 178 mg
Cholesterol 0 mg	Dietary Exchanges:
Sodium 77 mg	2½ other carbohydrate

Oatmeal-Raisin Drop Cookies

These soft and chewy cookies are quick and easy to make. In fact, you don't even need to use your mixer. Enjoy with a glass of fat-free milk.

SERVES 12
2 cookies per serving

Cooking spray
1½ cups uncooked quick-cooking oatmeal
½ cup whole-wheat flour
½ cup all-purpose flour
⅓ cup firmly packed light brown sugar
¼ cup sugar
1 teaspoon ground cinnamon
½ teaspoon baking powder
¼ teaspoon baking soda
⅛ teaspoon salt
⅓ cup unsweetened applesauce
1 large egg
1½ tablespoons light molasses
1 tablespoon canola or corn oil
1 teaspoon vanilla extract
½ cup raisins or dried sweetened cranberries

1. Preheat the oven to 350°F. Lightly spray two baking sheets with cooking spray. Set aside.

2. In a medium bowl, stir together the oatmeal, flours, sugars, cinnamon, baking powder, baking soda, and salt.

3. In a small bowl, whisk together the remaining ingredients except the raisins. Pour into the oatmeal mixture, stirring just until combined but no flour is visible. Stir in the raisins.

4. Drop the dough by tablespoons about 1½ inches apart on the baking sheets.

5. Bake for 12 to 14 minutes, or until the cookies begin to lightly brown. Transfer from the baking sheets to cooling racks. Let cool for at least 30 minutes.

6. Store leftover cookies in an airtight container, separating the layers with wax paper to keep the cookies from sticking together, for up to three days at room temperature. To store for up to six months, freeze baked cookies in airtight freezer containers or resealable freezer bags.

PER SERVING
Calories 164
Total Fat 2.5 g
Saturated Fat 0.5 g
Trans Fat 0.0 g
Polyunsaturated Fat 0.5 g
Monounsaturated Fat 1.0 g
Cholesterol 16 mg
Sodium 78 mg
Carbohydrates 33 g
Fiber 2 g
Sugars 17 g
Protein 4 g
Calcium 39 mg
Potassium 174 mg
Dietary Exchanges:
2 other carbohydrate, ½ fat

PART IV

Toolkit

DAILY SODIUM TRACKER

DATE	SERVING SIZE	SODIUM (MG)
breakfast		
	subtotal	
snack		
	subtotal	
lunch		
	subtotal	
snack		
	subtotal	
dinner		
	subtotal	
medications (if applicable)		
	total	

DAILY MENU PLANNER

DATE	CALORIES	SODIUM (MG)	FOOD GROUP*
breakfast			
		subtotal	
snack			
		subtotal	
lunch			
		subtotal	
snack			
		subtotal	
dinner			
		subtotal	
		total	

*The food groups can be abbreviated as follows: GR = Grain; VG = Vegetable; FR = Fruit; DA = Dairy; PRO = Protein source from seafood, lean meat or poultry, or other; LEG = Legume; FAT = Healthy fats and oils; NUT = Nut.

SODIUM-SAVVY SUBSTITUTIONS

REPLACE THIS . . .	SODIUM (MG)*	WITH THIS . . .	SODIUM (MG)*	FOR A SAVINGS OF . . .
breakfast				
1 fast-food breakfast sandwich	705	1 *Open-Face Breakfast Sandwich* (page 241)	295	410
1 large plain bagel with 2 tbsp cream cheese	635	1 plain thin bagel with 1 tbsp light tub cream cheese	310	325
2 slices pork bacon	370	2 slices turkey bacon	315	55
1 bakery zucchini-nut muffin	480	1 slice *Zucchini Quick Bread with Nuts and Fruit* (page 142)	110	370
8 oz mixed-vegetable juice	515	8 oz low-sodium mixed-vegetable juice	155	360
1 packet instant oatmeal, maple and brown sugar flavor	145	⅔ cup *Easy and Heart-y Oatmeal Mix* (page 240)	40	105
2 pancakes from mix and 2 tbsp pancake syrup	395	2 *Pancakes with Blueberry-Vanilla Sauce* (⅓ cup) (page 238)	305	90
lunch				
3 oz frozen chicken nuggets with 1 tbsp ketchup	410	3 oz *Crunchy Chicken Nuggets* (page 164) with 1 tbsp sauce	295	115
1 fast-food ¼-lb cheeseburger	900	1 fast-food ¼-lb hamburger	470	430
2 cups salad greens with 2 tbsp ranch dressing	290	2 cups salad greens with 2 tbsp *Ranch-Style Dressing with Green Onions* (page 224)	170	120
1 cup canned tomato-basil soup	735	1 cup *Roasted Tomato-Mushroom Bisque with Fresh Basil* (page 180)	225	510
¾ cup canned broccoli-cheese soup	360	¾ cup *Cheddar-Topped Broccoli Soup* (page 181)	160	200

REPLACE THIS . . .	SODIUM (MG)*	WITH THIS . . .	SODIUM (MG)*	FOR A SAVINGS OF . . .
dinner				
3 oz spaghetti with ½ cup bottled marinara sauce	480	3 oz whole-grain spaghetti with ½ cup *Mamma Mia Marinara* (page 215)	15	465
3 oz enhanced turkey with 2 tbsp instant brown gravy	530	3 oz *Roasted Turkey* (page 160) with 2 tbsp *Brown Gravy* (page 212)	165	365
3 oz chicken strips, seasoned fajita-style	725	3 oz grilled plain chicken strips with 2 tbsp *Spicy-Sweet Citrus-Cilantro Marinade* (page 214)	80	645
3 oz frozen fish fillets with ¼ cup cocktail sauce	665	3 oz *Crunchy Oven-Fried Fish Fillets* with 2 tbsp *Cocktail Sauce* (page 172)	380	285
1 individual frozen chicken potpie	1,070	1 cup *Chicken Phyllo Potpie* (page 162)	425	645
side dish				
½ cup macaroni and cheese	240	½ cup *Veggie Mac and Cheese* (page 192)	160	80
½ cup frozen creamed spinach	495	½ cup spinach cooked with 1 tsp olive oil and garlic	90	405
½ cup instant seasoned brown rice	345	½ cup instant unseasoned brown rice	5	340
½ cup canned corn	360	½ cup *Creamy Corn with Onions* (page 230)	130	230
½ cup scalloped potatoes from mix	445	½ cup *Scalloped Potato Casserole* (page 231)	165	280

***Sodium values represent the average of selected products and have been rounded to the nearest 5 mg. For recipes from this book, accurate sodium values are listed rounded to the nearest 5 mg.**

CONTINUED

REPLACE THIS . . .	SODIUM (MG)*	WITH THIS . . .	SODIUM (MG)*	FOR A SAVINGS OF . . .
dessert				
1 piece bakery carrot cake with cream cheese frosting	355	1 piece *Carrot Cake with Cream Cheese Frosting* (page 250)	95	260
½ cup instant lemon pudding, prepared	390	1 *Luscious Lemon Sponge Pudding* (page 248)	90	300
½ cup frozen apple cobbler	160	1 medium apple and 2 *Oatmeal-Raisin Drop Cookies* (page 252)	80	80
snack				
1 oz potato chips with ¼ cup bean dip	465	1 oz potato chips with ¼ cup *White Bean, Kalamata, and Basil Hummus* (page 204)	305	160
¼ cup salted peanuts	260	¼ cup dry-roasted peanuts, unsalted	0	260
1 oz tortilla chips and ¼ cup tomato salsa	450	8 *Italian-Style Tortilla Chips* (page 201) and ¼ cup *Fresh Tomato-Tomatillo Salsa* (page 210)	85	365

*Sodium values represent the average of selected products and have been rounded to the nearest 5 mg. For recipes from this book, accurate sodium values are listed rounded to the nearest 5 mg.

PRODUCT COMPARISON TRACKER

PRODUCT	SODIUM (MG) IN MY CURRENT CHOICE	COMPARABLE PRODUCT WITH LESS SODIUM	SODIUM (MG) IN NEW OPTION

NOTES:

SODIUM-SMART STAPLES

Keeping healthy staples on hand makes cooking healthy meals at home easier and more convenient. In fact, you'll be able to prepare most of the recipes in this book with the ingredients waiting in your well-stocked refrigerator, freezer, and pantry; for many other dishes, you'll need only a few additional items from the store.

FRESH

- onions
- garlic
- gingerroot
- lemons
- limes
- various chiles

FOR THE FRIDGE

- shredded Parmesan cheese
- fat-free or low-fat Cheddar and Monterey Jack cheese (lowest sodium available)
- low-fat mozzarella cheese
- eggs
- egg substitute
- light tub margarine or fat-free spray margarine
- light mayonnaise
- fat-free milk
- fat-free yogurt: plain, plain Greek, and sugar-free flavored

FOR THE FREEZER

- chicken breasts
- fish fillets
- assorted vegetables without added sauces
- brown rice
- lean steaks and chops
- extra-lean ground beef
- assorted fruits and berries

FOR THE PANTRY (nonperishables)

Rices (choose unseasoned)

- instant and/or regular brown rice
- instant and/or white rice

Beans and legumes

- no-salt-added canned kidney beans
- no-salt-added canned navy beans
- no-salt-added canned white beans
- no-salt-added canned black beans
- no-salt-added canned chickpeas
- dried beans, peas, and lentils

Pastas and grains

- assorted whole-grain and enriched pastas
- quick-cooking oatmeal
- whole-wheat couscous
- barley
- bulgur
- quinoa
- toasted wheat germ

Tomato products

- no-salt-added tomato sauce
- no-salt-added diced, stewed, crushed, and whole tomatoes
- no-salt-added tomato paste
- spaghetti sauces (lowest sodium available)

Dry goods

- flour—all-purpose, whole-wheat, white whole-wheat, bread, and cake
- sugar—granulated, light brown, dark brown, and confectioners'

- baking soda
- baking powder
- cornstarch
- cornmeal
- plain dry bread crumbs
- plain and plain whole-wheat panko (Japanese bread crumbs)
- active dry yeast
- salt-free instant bouillon—chicken and beef

Canned and bottled products

- fat-free, low-sodium broths
- low-sodium soups
- salmon (lowest sodium available) and very low sodium tuna in water
- no-salt-added canned vegetables
- fruits canned in water or their own juice
- 100 percent fruit juices
- unsweetened applesauce
- fat-free condensed milk
- fat-free evaporated milk
- roasted red bell peppers
- olives
- green chiles
- garlic—minced, chopped, or whole
- gingerroot, minced

Cooking oils

- cooking sprays
- canola or corn oil
- olive oil
- toasted sesame oil

Miscellaneous

- peanut butter (lowest sodium available)
- all-fruit spreads
- honey
- maple syrup
- molasses
- unsalted nuts, such as almonds, walnuts, peanuts, and pecans
- dried fruits, such as raisins, cranberries, and apricots
- seeds, such as sesame, poppy, caraway, pumpkin (unsalted), and sunflower (unsalted)

CONDIMENTS
(choose lowest sodium available)

- vinegars, such as plain rice, cider, balsamic, red wine, and plain rice wine
- mustards
- no-salt-added ketchup
- hoisin sauce
- red hot-pepper sauce
- salsa
- soy sauce
- teriyaki sauce
- Worcestershire sauce
- barbecue sauce

SPICES AND SEASONINGS

- dried herbs including oregano, basil, thyme, rosemary, dillweed, parsley, sage, and summer savory
- garlic powder
- onion powder
- chili powder
- curry powder
- dry mustard
- crushed red pepper flakes
- black pepper
- cayenne
- salt-free seasoning blends, such as Italian and all-purpose
- ground spices, such as cinnamon, ginger, nutmeg, allspice, cumin, paprika, and smoked paprika
- salt
- vanilla extract

FOOD GROUPS AND SUGGESTED SERVINGS

For each basic food group, the following chart lists the average numbers of recommended servings, which are based on daily calorie intake. The number of servings that is right for you will vary depending on your caloric needs. When shopping, compare nutrition facts panels and look for the products that are lowest in sodium, saturated fat, trans fat, and cholesterol, and that don't have added sugars.

SERVING RECOMMENDATIONS BY CALORIE LEVEL

FOOD GROUP	1,600 CALORIES	2,000 CALORIES	2,600 CALORIES	SAMPLE SERVING SIZES
vegetables Eat a variety of colors and types.	3 to 4 servings per day	4 to 5 servings per day	5 to 6 servings per day	1 cup raw leafy vegetable ½ cup cut-up raw or cooked nonleafy vegetable ½ cup vegetable juice
fruits Eat a variety of colors and types.	4 servings per day	4 to 5 servings per day	5 to 6 servings per day	1 medium fruit ¼ cup dried fruit ½ cup fresh, frozen, or canned fruit ½ cup fruit juice
fiber-rich whole grains Choose whole grains for at least half your servings.	6 servings per day	6 to 8 servings per day	10 to 11 servings per day	1 slice bread 1 oz dry cereal (check nutrition label for cup measurements) ½ cup cooked rice, pasta, or cereal
fat-free, 1% fat, and low-fat dairy products Choose fat-free when possible but compare sodium levels.	2 to 3 servings per day	2 to 3 servings per day	3 servings per day	1 cup milk 1 cup yogurt 1½ oz cheese

FOOD GROUP	1,600 CALORIES	2,000 CALORIES	2,600 CALORIES	SAMPLE SERVING SIZES
fish Choose varieties rich in omega-3 fatty acids.	6 to 7 oz (cooked) per week	6 to 7 oz (cooked) per week	6 to 7 oz (cooked) per week	3 to 3½ oz cooked fish, such as salmon and trout
lean meats and skinless poultry Choose lean and extra-lean.	3 oz (cooked) per day	3 to 6 oz (cooked) per day	6 oz (cooked) per day	3 oz cooked poultry or meat
legumes, nuts, and seeds Choose unsalted products.	3 servings per week	4 to 5 servings per week	1 serving per day	½ cup dried beans or peas ⅓ cup or 1½ oz nuts 2 tbsp peanut butter 2 tbsp or ½ oz seeds
fats and oils Use liquid vegetable oil and spray or light tub margarines most often. Choose products with the lowest amount of sodium.	2 servings per day	2 to 3 servings per day	2 to 3 servings per day	1 tsp light tub margarine 1 tbsp light mayonnaise 1 tsp vegetable oil 1 tbsp regular or 2 tbsp low-fat salad dressing (fat-free dressing does not count as a serving but does contain calories)

Source: Adapted from the DASH (Dietary Approaches to Stop Hypertension) eating plan developed by the National Heart, Lung, and Blood Institute, National Institutes of Health.

SODIUM-FREE FLAVORING SUGGESTIONS

breads	Anise, caraway seeds, cardamom, citrus zest, fennel, dried fruits, poppy seeds, sesame seeds
desserts	Anise, caraway seeds, cardamom, cinnamon, cloves, coriander, ginger, mace, mint, nutmeg, dry-roasted unsalted nuts, poppy seeds, vanilla and other extracts
entrées	
beef	Allspice, bay leaf, bell pepper, cayenne, cumin, curry powder, garlic, fresh horseradish, marjoram, fresh mushrooms, dry mustard, onion, pepper, rosemary, sage, thyme, table wine
pork	Apple, applesauce, caraway seeds, cherries, cinnamon, cloves, fennel, garlic, ginger, mint, onion, oranges or orange juice, peaches, sage, savory, table wine
poultry	Basil, bay leaf, bell pepper, cinnamon, citrus fruits, cranberries, curry powder, garlic, kiwifruit, lemon juice, lemon pepper, mace, marjoram, fresh mushrooms, onion, oregano, paprika, parsley, rosemary, saffron, sage, savory, sesame, tarragon, thyme, table wine
seafood	Allspice, basil, bay leaf, bell pepper, cayenne, curry powder, cumin, fennel, garlic, lemon juice, mace, marjoram, mint, fresh mushrooms, dry mustard, onion, paprika, saffron, sage, sesame seeds, tarragon, thyme, turmeric, table wine
salads	Basil, chervil, coriander, dillweed, lemon juice, mint, dry mustard, oregano, parsley, rosemary, sage, savory, sesame seeds, turmeric, vinegar, watercress
vegetables	
asparagus	Garlic, lemon juice, onion, dry-roasted sesame seeds
beans, dried	Caraway seeds, cloves, cumin, mint, savory, tarragon, thyme
beets	Anise, caraway seeds, fennel, ginger, orange juice, savory
carrots	Anise, cinnamon, cloves, mint, sage, tarragon
corn	Allspice, bell pepper, cumin, pimiento, tomato
cucumbers	Chives, dillweed, garlic, vinegar
green beans	Dillweed, lemon juice, marjoram, nutmeg, pimiento
greens	Garlic, lemon juice, onion, pepper, vinegar
peas	Allspice, bell pepper, mint, fresh mushrooms, onions, parsley, sage, savory
potatoes	Bell pepper, chives, dillweed, garlic, onion, pimiento, saffron
spinach	Garlic, lemon juice, vinegar
squash	Allspice, brown sugar, cinnamon, cloves, fennel, ginger, mace, nutmeg, onion, savory
tomatoes	Allspice, basil, garlic, marjoram, onion, oregano, sage, savory, tarragon, thyme

WARNING SIGNS OF HEART ATTACK AND STROKE

Heart attack and stroke are life-and-death emergencies—every second counts. If you see or have any of the listed symptoms, immediately call 9-1-1 or your emergency response number. Not all these signs occur in every heart attack or stroke. Sometimes they go away and return. If some occur, get help fast.

HEART ATTACK

Some heart attacks are sudden and intense, but most start slowly, with mild pain or discomfort. Watch for these warning signs:

- **Chest discomfort.** Most heart attacks involve discomfort in the center of the chest that lasts more than a few minutes, or that goes away and comes back. It can feel like uncomfortable pressure, squeezing, fullness, or pain.
- **Discomfort in other areas of the upper body.** Symptoms can include pain or discomfort in one or both arms or in the back, neck, jaw, or stomach.
- **Shortness of breath.** This may occur with or without chest discomfort.
- **Other signs.** These may include breaking out in a cold sweat, nausea, or light-headedness.

The most common heart attack symptom for both women and men is chest pain or discomfort. Women, however, are more likely to experience some of the other common symptoms, particularly shortness of breath, nausea/vomiting, and back or jaw pain.

STROKE

Stroke is a medical emergency. Time lost is brain cells lost, so don't delay—get help right away. Learn to recognize the warning signs:

- Sudden numbness or weakness of the face, arm, or leg, especially on one side of the body
- Sudden confusion, trouble speaking, or difficulty understanding
- Sudden trouble seeing in one or both eyes
- Sudden trouble walking, dizziness, or loss of balance or coordination
- Sudden severe headache with no known cause

general index

Note: Page numbers in **bold type** refer to charts.

recipe index